Praise for *The 3-Hour Diet™*

"Thi

—Davi
col

"Combinin   se's
revolution   lim

—Carol Brooks, editor in chief, *First for Women* magazine

"Jorge Cruise has identified a fundamental tenet of successful weight
loss—that how you eat is just as important as what you eat. In short,
his book is an essential tool for those seeking lifelong weight loss
and maintenance."

**—Lisa Sanders, MD, Yale University School of Medicine,
author of *The Perfect Fit Diet***

"The 3-Hour Diet™ offers a simple nutrition prescription: how
often and how much to control your hunger, enjoy your food, and
improve your health. You can't get much better than that!"

**—Leslie Bonci, MPH, RD, LDN, director of sports medicine
nutrition, University of Pittsburgh Medical Center, and
nutritionist for the Pittsburgh Steelers**

"Jorge Cruise brings a new dimension to the world of weight loss—
empowering and giving you the tools to lose weight by making
simple changes in how and when you eat. This technique can
help make all the difference."

**—Fred Pescatore, MD, author of *The Hamptons Diet* and
former associate medical director at the Atkins® Center**

"Feel like pasta for dinner? Not a problem. Some toast with those eggs?
Bring it on. With Jorge's 3-Hour Diet™, eating great and losing
weight has never been this simple."

—Jacqui Stafford, *Shape* magazine

OTHER BOOKS BY JORGE CRUISE:

Collins gem

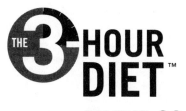

THE 3-HOUR DIET™

ON THE GO

Set Your
Metabolism in
Motion™ and Lose
Belly Fat First!

JORGE CRUISE
AOL's Diet Coach

Collins
An Imprint of HarperCollins*Publishers*

HarperCollins books may be purchased for educational,
business, or sales promotional use. For information, please
write: Special Markets Department, HarperCollins Publishers,
10 East 53rd Street, New York, NY 10022.

FIRST EDITION

Designed by Ellen Cipriano and Lorie Pagnozzi

Client photographs courtesy JorgeCruise.com, Inc.

ISBN-10: 0-06-079319-8   ISBN-13: 978-0-06-079319-7

06 07 08 09 WBC/WOR 10 9 8 7 6 5 4

Contents

SIX Bonus Resources

ACKNOWLEDGMENTS

From the first day I started the adventure of writing the 3-Hour Diet™ books, it has been the millions of women and men who have trusted me with their health and their weight loss who have continually inspired me and kept me searching for a better way to change the way the world eats. To all of you, I express my undying appreciation and gratitude.

To my wife, Heather, and my amazing little boy, a bundle of life and energy, Parker—coming home to you each day is the greatest joy of my life. You make it all worthwhile, and I consider myself the luckiest man in the world to have both of you in my life.

I always must thank Oprah Winfrey for

launching my career as an author, and because she serves as a constant inspiration to me and to millions of others whose lives she touches with her compassion and commitment to excellence.

To Ben Gage, president of my company, my friend and trusted advisor. With your steadfast leadership and support we are continuing to build a company and the strategic relationships that will carry the message of the 3-Hour Diet™ to millions of people around the world.

Of course, my heartfelt thanks go out to my special friends and expert advisors Lisa Sharkey, Carol Brooks, Michele Hatty, Liz Brody, and Jacqui Stafford for their constant support and insightful advice on what people truly want when it comes to dieting.

To our marketing partners for the 3-Hour Diet™ Revolution—Rick and Mike Anderson of PurFoods, creators of the 3-Hour Diet™ At Home Fresh Food Delivery Service; and Al Czap, Scott Sensenbrenner, and Phil Luetkemyer of Thorne Research, Inc., creators of the 3-Hour Diet™ Meal Replacement products.

Russell Speck and our entire IT team at eJungle who are always there when we need them, day or night, to keep the online pieces of the 3-Hour Diet™ humming.

To Alisa Bauman, whose editorial eye has helped me shape this and my many other books—thank you.

To my advisory circle: Thank you Halle Elbling, MS, RD; Vanessa Aldaz, MPH, RD; Linda Spangle, RN, MA; Janette J. Gray, MD; Cory Baker, CPT, NASM; Chef Bernard Guillas; Andrew Roorda, MD; and Jade Beutler, supplement expert. I am so grateful for your time, efforts, and friendship. Thanks so much!

Everyone at HarperCollins, thank you so much for your continued support of the 3-Hour Diet™ and the launch of our books. Special thank you's to Jane Friedman, Brian Murray, Joe Tessitore, Kathy Huck (the most patient editor in publishing), George Bick, Shelby Meizlik, Jill Goldstein, Tara Cibelli, and everyone else at this amazing company.

Finally, and most important, to my inner team at JorgeCruise.com, Inc. Phyllis McClanahan, Jenn Anderson, Heidi Hageman, Cory

Baker, thank you for making my job so much easier with your passion, commitment, and supreme effort in support of my vision for the 3-Hour Diet™.

W ELCOME TO THE

Dear Friend,

Welcome to a new revolution in eating! If you are like me, you need a healthy, truly enjoyable, and *realistic way* to shed pounds and maintain your ideal weight.

Well, for the past 10 years finding that way has been my primary focus. I have been privileged to work with more than 3 million online clients and to listen to their requests and feedback. Everything I learned reinforced what I already knew. You see, I used to be an overweight kid and young man. What I learned is weight loss had to be made easy. That meant no deprivation, no counting calories, no counting points, and no counting carbs. We are all too busy. If that sounds like you, then you've come to the right place, because what you now hold in your hands is a new secret weapon.

I am thrilled to share with you my newest breakthrough in healthy living. The 3-Hour Diet™ is truly a revolution in eating and dieting. It will transform your health and waistline in the most simple and enjoyable manner. Bottom line, eat the right foods every 3 hours

3-HOUR DIET™

and you will lose weight—starting with belly fat first! The 3-Hour Diet™ is about uncovering the buried concept of *timing*—the fact that *when* you eat is critical to weight loss.

In this all-new 3-Hour Diet™ book get ready to discover the most delicious meals, snacks, treats, and drinks for eating *on the go*. This portable guide presents you with more than 600 "at-your-fingertip" options to help you achieve and maintain the body of your dreams—without having to cook! Whether you're out at a restaurant, hitting the drive-through, stopping for gas, or having less than 5 minutes to eat, this pocket guide will get you through the day and keep you from slipping.

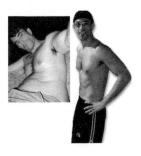

So, as you begin the 3-Hour Diet™, make a

commitment to put aside any past beliefs or convictions that may be limiting you, and, most important, to take care of your mind, body, and spirit at the deepest levels. The result is that you will not only feel better and have more energy, but you will experience a new sense of excitement and joy in your life.

Congratulations on making the commitment to take action and achieve the extraordinary health you deserve!

Your friend and coach,

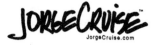

JorgeCruise.com

Jorge Cruise
AOL's DIET COACH
AND THE CREATOR OF 3HOURDIET.NET

P.S. *This practical guide complements the original* New York Times *best-selling 3-Hour Diet™, which contains more than 50 homemade recipes. If you can spare some time to enjoy cooking, you won't want to miss that book. But with this convenient guide, no cooking is necessary.*

ONE

QUICK GUIDE TO
THE 3-HOUR DIET™

The 3-Hour Diet™ is about uncovering the buried concept of *timing*—the fact that *when* you eat is critical to weight loss. By eating every 3 hours you'll constantly *Set Your Metabolism in Motion™* and lose 2 pounds every week starting with belly fat first. You will never have to count calories or ban any foods, including carbs.

So how does the 3-Hour Diet™ work exactly? The answer is found in what I call *Time-Based Nutrition™*. It's the future of effective nutrition. No more low-carb dieting. No more fad dieting. *Time-Based Nutrition*™ is a brand-new category of dieting. It's the power of combining smart eating with smart timing. Yes, timing. You see, the secret to losing weight and keeping it off has to do with much more than *what* you eat, it's also *when* you eat.

Why every 3 hours? Countless research studies confirm the power of eating every 3 hours. What specifically happens if you wait more than 3 hours to eat? Well, after 3 hours your body passes a tipping point and launches its natural "starvation protection mechanism," or SPM. When your SPM is switched on, your body preserves the most calorie-rich tissue in the body to ensure your survival. That tissue is body fat. But there's even more bad news. **It's critical to know that anytime you allow more than 3 hours to pass between meals, your body preserves body fat and begins to *cannibalize* precious fat-burning muscle.** Yes, by waiting more than 3 hours to eat you lose muscle tissue.

Why is losing lean muscle devastating to your health? Lean muscle tissue is your *metabolism*.

Bottom line: it burns fat and thus sets your metabolism in motion. Lean muscle tissue manages how many calories you burn while doing nothing, whether you're resting on the couch, driving your car, sitting at the computer, or even when sleeping in your bed. Each pound of muscle burns approximately 50 calories every day doing absolutely nothing. Lose just 5 pounds of muscle and your metabolism burns 250 fewer calories a day. In the course of just one year that will equal 26 pounds of new fat—no wonder dieting has been so difficult! Make sure to visit 3hourdiet.net to get a free profile to help you determine how much muscle you've lost.

There is one more devastating consequence of not eating every 3 hours: *increased cortisol levels*. What exactly is cortisol? It's a stress hormone that is closely associated with abdominal fat. The good news is that medical research has shown that eating every 3 hours helps reduce levels of cortisol, and that is the key to losing belly fat first. For more on this, make sure to read chapter 5 of the original *3-Hour Diet™*.

Okay, so what are the smartest foods to eat? The best foods are the foods *you* love in the proper serving. Yes, the secret is choosing the right amounts of the foods you enjoy. My core philosophy is that there are no bad foods, just bad timing and unhealthy portions. Banning the foods you love will guarantee failure. For this reason I created the 3-Hour Plate™ in the original *3-Hour Diet™*. It shows you how to avoid calorie counting and saves your precious time by helping you stay organized with a *visual* system.

But here's the best news about this little book: since it is for people on the go, you won't even need to use the 3-Hour Plate™ to eat the right foods. My nutrition team and I have done all the work for you! Yes, we have researched your favorite fast-food joints, family restaurants, meal replacement bars, and even a few more special things to bring you the ultimate guidebook to enjoying the 3-Hour Diet™ with no hassles and, best of all, no cooking!

That is why you will **love** this easy-to-use guide.

Why Do Low-Carb Diets Make You Fat?

In the short term, low-carb diets absolutely lead to weight loss. In the long term, you will end up gaining the weight back and you may find that you have added new pounds, too. The bottom line is this: Anytime you go on a high-protein diet, which is low in carbs, you begin to lose up to 25 percent of your lean muscle. Lean muscle tissue, as I shared with you earlier, is essential for an active fat-burning metabolism.

Specifically, low-carb diets erode muscle in three major ways:

A) Low-carb diets deplete the sugar (glycogen) stored in your muscles.

B) Low-carb diets flush water out of your muscles.

C) Low-carb diets can cause fatigue and/or depression, which leads to a sedentary lifestyle. When you don't move, you lose muscle faster.

Finally, if you deprive yourself of carbs, you will eventually binge on them. I have worked with 3 million online clients at 3hourdiet.net and they've told me about this time and time again. It's practically a fact. Deprivation leads to bingeing and long-term failure.

Basic rules for the 3-Hour Diet™

1. Eat Every 3 Hours

Frequent meals will help keep your metabolism running smoothly for the whole day. The key is eating throughout the day, with 3 hours between meals. In other words, if you eat breakfast at 7 a.m., have a snack at 10 a.m., eat lunch at 1 p.m., have another snack at 4 p.m., and finally eat dinner at 7 p.m., you can finish off the day by having your treat, which may be eaten with dinner or anytime within the next 3 hours before bed. It's up to you! This is a perfect eating schedule, and I strongly recommend you closely follow this time pattern.

2. Bend and Flex

Is your schedule unique? Not a problem! The 3-Hour Diet™ is designed to bend and flex with your daily schedule *for stress-free dieting*. For ideal results I recommend you stick as closely to the plan as possible, but, more important, stick to these three basic principles:

1. Eat absolutely as close to every 3 hours as possible
2. Eat the 3 recommended meals, 2 snacks, and treat each day
3. Eat breakfast within 1 hour of rising

Here are some sample plans to help you understand how the 3-Hour Diet™ can adapt to your schedule with ease:

FOR THE *VERY LATE* RISER:

Noon: Brunch
3 p.m.: Snack
6 p.m.: Lunch (early dinner) AND snack*
9 p.m.: Dinner AND treat*

*NOTE: Combining snacks and treats with meals is Okay!

FOR THE LATE RISER:

10 a.m.: Breakfast
1 p.m.: Lunch*
4 p.m.: Snack
7 p.m.: Dinner
9 p.m.: Treat AND snack

*NOTE: Snack skipped between lunch and dinner, and combined with treat

FOR THE EARLY BIRD:

4 a.m.: Breakfast
7 a.m.: Snack
10 a.m.: Lunch
1 p.m.: Snack
4 p.m.: Dinner
7 p.m.: Treat

*NOTE: You're up early, so chances are you will be going to bed early, too.
Eating every 3 hours should not interrupt your schedule.

3. Select the Right Number of Calories

You should consume 1,450 calories a day. Although I've done all of the calorie counting for you, I thought you'd like to see how those calories break down into meals and snacks.

Sample day

7 a.m.

Breakfast—400 calories of balanced nutrients

10 a.m.

Snack A—100 calories

1 p.m.

Lunch—400 calories of balanced nutrients

4 p.m.

Snack B—100 calories

7 p.m.

Dinner—400 calories of balanced nutrients

10 p.m.

Treat—50 calories

NOTE: Visit 3hourdiet.net for more examples.

Depending on your current weight, you may need to adjust this plan according to your personal metabolism. Assuming you weigh less than 200 pounds, the above plan will work for you. However, if you weigh more, make the following changes:

- 200 to 249 pounds: double your snack size to 200 calories

- 250 to 299 pounds: triple your snack size to 300 calories

- 300 pounds or more: raise your snack size to 400 calories OR add another meal

As your weight drops, adjust to the next calorie selection to continue losing 2 pounds a week. If you weigh less than 150 pounds and are short in stature (under 5'3"), 1,450 calories may be too much food for you. You can solve this simply by cutting your breakfast in half and eating only 200 calories during this meal, for a total daily intake of 1,250 calories. See page 85 of the original *3-Hour Diet™* for even more details.

Two Secrets to Ensuring Your Success

- Secret #1: Stay organized
- Secret #2: Avoid emotional eating

How will you stay organized? Your secret weapon will be what I call the 3-Hour Timeline™. Here's how you create your timeline: each day you will need a piece of paper and a pen (see page 13). On your sheet of paper draw a long vertical line with an arrow pointing down. This line will represent your day. At the top of the paper, draw one small horizontal line that crosses the vertical line. This will be your breakfast. Continue with five more horizontal lines to represent your snack, lunch, second snack, and dinner. Finally, add one last horizontal line (your sixth line down) for your treat. Your treat may be eaten with dinner.

Next, on the far left, indicate the time you choose to eat each meal, snack, and treat. It's that simple.

Now for the fun part! On the right, just pick

your favorite foods from the lists on pages 22 to 107.

Don't forget to include eight circles at the bottom to represent eight glasses of water. Although water is not a food, it is essential for weight loss. Why? Research has shown that drinking one 16-ounce glass of water will boost your metabolism by 30 percent within 40 minutes and will keep it elevated for more than an hour. My recommendation is to drink 1 ounce of water for every 2 pounds of body weight. If you weigh 160 pounds, aim for 80 ounces. Always make sure to drink the cleanest water you can find. My tip to my online clients is to try Penta® Water. It undergoes a 13-step, 11-hour purification process designed to remove every possible impurity including arsenic, bacteria, chlorine, chromium-6, fluoride, lead, MTBE, and pesticides.

And if you are looking for the easiest way to create your 3-Hour Timeline™, make sure to visit 3HourDiet.net to create customized daily plans in a pinch.

A Sample 3-Hour Timeline™:

7 AM	Breakfast	- Lean Pocket - ½ cup cottage cheese + fruit
10 AM	Snack	- Dannon - Light 'N Fit Smoothie
1 PM	Lunch	- McDonald's Cheeseburger - Side salad
4 PM	Snack	- Granola Bar (Low-Fat)
7 PM	Dinner	- Healthy Choice Tuna Casserole - Side salad
10 PM	Treat	- Reese's Peanut Butter Cup

Now, to stay motivated, I highly recommend you take a "before" photo right now. I know you may be thinking, "Jorge, I don't want to take a picture. I don't like how I look." Believe me, I didn't want to take the picture of me that you probably saw on page xiii of this book. But it's important! Taking a picture before you start the program symbolizes that you're about to change. It signifies that you are finally taking action—that it's time for a new beginning. More important, you'll love it when you have lost the weight and have a new, fantastic photo to compare it to. You'll be amazed by your changes. Make sure to e-mail your photos and success story to us at success@3hourdiet.net, and I will e-mail you back. You might even appear in a future book or on my 3hourdiet.net site.

Additionally, what I would like you to do next is write down your *goal weight* and target date on the next page. Your target date is the anticipated date on which you will reach your goal. Here is how that works: All you need to do is subtract your current weight from your goal weight and that will give you a number. Say it's 50 pounds. And if it's 50 pounds, you simply divide it by the number 2. Why 2? Because on average you will be losing 2 pounds every week. So there it is, the number of weeks it will take you to achieve your goal. Get out your calendar and circle that wonderful date because this is going to become your new birth date—the date you finally begin to live the life you have been dreaming of!

How to Avoid Emotional Eating

This is a subject that is almost always overlooked in weight-loss plans. Well, not here. What exactly is emotional eating? Here's the big answer: ***It's eating anytime you are not hungry.*** It's that simple and yet it's the #1 saboteur of almost all dieters.

I used to be an emotional eater. The truth is, as a kid and young man, food was my best friend and I turned to it anytime I felt an emotional challenge. My parents never taught me healthy ways to manage these kinds of challenges. So I simply coped with my problems via food. It was my solution to every difficult emotion I encountered.

How did I overcome it? In the original *3-Hour Diet™* I shared my People Solution™ plan, which explains how to eliminate emotional eating. For now, here's my super-quick explanation.

If you feel you are about to eat emotionally, ask yourself the following question:

"Is this what I really need?"

Odds are (if you are about to eat for emotional reasons) the answer to the question is . . .

No!

But you might be saying to yourself, *"I want to feel better . . . I am sad, I am depressed. I am lonely, I am angry, I am stressed, I am overwhelmed, I need to feel better now, etc. . . . "*

Here's the trick: instead of using food yet again as a crutch that will later make you feel guilty and of course make you even more overweight, use something you have not used in years.

Do you know what this is?

YOU.

Yep, you need to become your own best friend—fast. You need to *nurture yourself* in this time of need. How do you effectively nurture yourself? How do you do it quickly? How can you fill yourself up with something more powerful and stronger than food?

The solution is simple. *You need to* **see** *your desired future now.*

My 3-Hour Diet™
Success Contract

Filling out this contract will help keep you accountable to your goals. Make three copies and give them to three trusted friends who will support and motivate you in your journey to success.

Name: _____

Today's date: _____

I am going to weigh this many pounds: _____

By this date: _____

_____
Signature

Photocopy this contract and place on your refrigerator. Join 3hourdiet.net for support and to stay accountable.

YES, you need to see it now. You need to see the ideal you. Now. See yourself walking as a confident person. See yourself in control, and being decisive with yourself, friends, and family about your meal and food decisions.

Envision how happy you are from living with a slim, sexy, and firm body for years. See yourself standing tall with your shoulders back and chest out. See your smile. See yourself enjoying your lifelong dream of visiting a faraway land, marrying your soul mate, or playing with your kids or grandkids.

Positive visualizations are critical to your success if you are an emotional eater. In fact, you never lose the weight if your emotions control you. This is why on pages 135 to 142 I have included a week's worth of visualizations. And for more support on overcoming emotional eating, join 3HourDiet.net.

How to Use This Book

This book is divided into five main sections that will give you exactly what you need to select your meals, snacks, and treats, no matter where you are when it's time to eat.

If it's time for breakfast and you want to know what to eat on the go, turn to chapter 2. If you're looking for lunch or dinner with no preparation, check out chapter 3. To find tasty snacks that are easy to grab at a vending machine or mini-mart, go to chapter 4. For delicious treats that'll satisfy your chocolate craving, turn to chapter 5. If you don't want to eat "on the go," then make sure to pick up a copy of my original *3-Hour Diet™* book. It has more than fifty recipes and a built-in meal planner.

Keep this book in your car, briefcase, or purse. Anytime you find yourself asking, "What should I eat?" just flip to the appropriate section and find all of your 3-Hour Diet™–approved options. Whether you need to grab fast food, restaurant food, "gas station gourmet," or a meal-replacement bar or shake, it's all right here. Eating smart when you're on the go is the key to your success, and this handbook will help you do it right!

As a bonus, the resources in chapter 6 will give you the extra edge. I've included success stories from my clients to provide you with inspiration, along with their secrets to success. You'll also find visualizations for an instant pick-me-up when you're having a tough time staying dedicated to your weight-loss goal. In addition, I've included a guide to drinking alcohol on the 3-Hour Diet™ and a guide to dining at special events, making eating every 3 hours the realistic solution you have been searching for.

Okay, now that you understand the importance of timing and the secrets to ensure your success, it's time to use this book and begin losing 2 pounds every week, starting with belly fat first! Remember: eating equals enjoyment and this guide will enable you to choose from all your favorite "on the go" foods. Finally, no banned foods!

You hold the key to the lifetime of health you've been searching for. Get ready to Set Your Metabolism in Motion™ and get out there and enjoy life!

TWO

BREAKFAST ON THE GO

ALL MEALS ARE APPROXIMATELY 400 CALORIES.

Breakfast Overview

Breakfast:
<u>Fast Food</u> Meal Options

These selections are the healthiest options that approximately meet the 3-Hour Plate™ criteria.

Arby's® Sourdough Egg'n Swiss Sandwich

- Add fruit.*

Arby's® Ham Biscuit

- Add fruit.*

Arby's® Bacon Biscuit

- Add fruit.*

Chick-fil-A® Chick-n-minis™

- Order the 4 count.
- Add fruit.*

---

*See pages 98–103 for a list of 3-Hour Diet™–approved fruits and vegetables.

Del Taco® Breakfast Burrito

- Add 1% milk.

Hardee's Frisco Breakfast Sandwich

- Add fruit.*

Hardee's Hash Rounds (medium)

- Add Breakfast Ham and fruit.*

Hardee's Made from Scratch Biscuit

- Add Breakfast Ham and a piece of fruit.*

Jack in the Box® Breakfast Jack®

- Add 2% milk and fruit.*

Jamba Juice® Berry Fulfilling™ (16 oz.)

- Jamba Juice® provides a scoop of
  supplement off their menu. Choose

---

*See pages 98–103 for a list of 3-Hour Diet™-approved fruits
and vegetables.

protein AND take 4 flaxseed oil capsules
or 1 teaspoon flaxseed oil.

Jamba Juice® Mango Mantra™ (16 oz.)

- Jamba Juice® provides a scoop of
  supplement off their menu. Choose
  protein AND take 4 flaxseed oil capsules
  or 1 teaspoon flaxseed oil.

Jamba Juice® Strawberry Nirvana™ (16 oz.)

- Jamba Juice® provides a scoop of
  supplement off their menu. Choose
  protein AND take 4 flaxseed oil capsules
  or 1 teaspoon flaxseed oil.

Jamba Juice® Tropical Awakening™ (16 oz.)

- Jamba Juice® provides a scoop of
  supplement off their menu. Choose
  protein AND take 4 flaxseed oil capsules
  or 1 teaspoon flaxseed oil.

*See pages 98–103 for a list of 3-Hour Diet™–approved fruits
and vegetables.

McDonald's® Egg McMuffin®

- Add 1% milk and fruit.*

McDonald's® Sausage Burrito

- Add fruit* (apple is available at McDonald's).

SUBWAY® Vegetable and Egg (breakfast sandwich)

- Ask for EXTRA veggies.

SUBWAY® Bacon & Egg (breakfast sandwich) on Deli Round

- Add fruit.*

SUBWAY® Cheese and Egg (breakfast sandwich) on Deli Round

- Add fruit.*

---

*See pages 98–103 for a list of 3-Hour Diet™–approved fruits and vegetables.

SUBWAY® Steak & Egg (breakfast sandwich) on Deli Round

- Add fruit.*

SUBWAY® Vegetable and Egg (breakfast sandwich) on Deli Round

- Add fruit* OR ask for EXTRA veggies.

SUBWAY® Western Egg (breakfast sandwich) on Deli Round

- Add fruit.*

SUBWAY® Vegetable and Egg Omelet

- Add fruit* OR ask for EXTRA veggies.

*See pages 98–103 for a list of 3-Hour Diet™–approved fruits and vegetables.

Breakfast:
Restaurant Meal Options

These selections are the healthiest options that fulfill the criteria of the 3-Hour Plate™.

Coco's Bakery® à la carte menu

Select items according to the 3-Hour Plate™. You can use these options as a reference to your choices.

Option 1

1 egg, any style
1 cup of yogurt
⅓ cup granola
½ plate of fruit

Option 2

3 eggs, poached
1 piece of toast, preferably whole wheat
Pat of butter
½ plate fruit

Einstein Bros.® Bagel Frittata Egg Sandwich

Choose one of the following choices of frittata; any bagel will do. Don't forget to add a piece of fruit AND split the frittata with a friend or save the other half for later.

- Plain with Cheddar.
- Thick Cut Smoked Bacon & Cheddar.
- Black Forest Ham & Swiss.
- Turkey Sausage & Cheddar.

Denny's® Veggie Egg Beaters® Omelette (Fit Fare™ Menu)

- Add tomato juice.

Denny's® à la carte menu

Select items according to the 3-Hour Plate™. The following options are available on the Denny's® menu and can be used as a reference for your choices.

Option 1

1 egg, any style

1 Grilled Honey Ham Slice

1 piece of toast, dry, preferably whole wheat

½ grapefruit

Option 2

Two Buttermilk Pancakes with Sugar-Free Maple-
   Flavored Syrup

1 egg, poached

1 Grilled Honey Ham Slice

Order of grapes

Option 3

Cold cereal with milk

1 egg, any style

Glass of tomato juice

IHOP® Build Your Own Omelette

Tip for Building

2 eggs (or 6 egg whites)

1 ounce cheese or 1 ounce ham (or other meat)

Add cup of orange juice or a healthy serving of veggies
or fruit*.

Mimi's Café® Two AA Large Egg Breakfast

- Order Egg Beaters®.
- Substitute sliced tomatoes for the potatoes.
- Wheat toast, dry.

*See pages 98–103 for a list of 3-Hour Diet™–approved fruits
and vegetables.

Breakfast:
Frozen Meal Options

These selections are the healthiest options that fulfill the criteria of the 3-Hour Plate™.

Amy's® Apple, Strawberry or Strawberry & Cream Cheese Toaster Pops (1)

- Add 3 eggs, any style.

Amy's® Tofu Scramble in a Pocket Sandwich

- Add fruit.*

Easy Omelets® Omelet, Cheddar Flavor

- Add fruit.*

Eggo® Nutri-Grain® Low-Fat Blueberry Waffles (2)

- Add a fluffy mixture of 2 eggs (or 6 egg whites) scrambled with water and 1 ounce

---

*See pages 98–103 for a list of 3-Hour Diet™–approved fruits and vegetables.

of the cheese of your choice. Top it off
with a piece of fruit or a cup of berries
and enjoy! Note: When preparing eggs in a
nonstick skillet, use cooking spray if
necessary.

Eggo® Nutri-Grain® Low-Fat Waffles (2)

- Spread 1 teaspoon of peanut butter on the
  waffles. Prepare 3 slices of lean turkey
  bacon and add a glass of 1% milk or ¼
  cup of low-fat cottage cheese. Don't forget
  to add the fruit and have a delicious
  breakfast.

Hot Pockets® Ham & Cheese

- Add fruit* and 6 ounces of 1% milk.

Lean Pockets® Sausage, Egg & Low Fat Cheese (1)

- Add ½ cup of low-fat cottage cheese and
  fruit.*

* See pages 98–103 for a list of 3-Hour Diet™–approved fruits
and vegetables.

Morningstar Farms™ Veggie Breakfast Sausage Patty

- Add 1 cup orange juice.

WeightWatchers® SMART ONES® English Muffin Sandwich (1)

- Add fruit.*

*See pages 98–103 for a list of 3-Hour Diet™–approved fruits and vegetables.

Breakfast:
Bars/Shakes Meal Options

The following are the easiest breakfast options for when you truly have no time. There are two options. Option 1 combines a 200-calorie bar with a 200-calorie yogurt from well-known brands. Although they do not precisely fit the nutritional requirements of the 3-Hour Diet™, when combined they get the job done. **Option 2 combines a 200-calorie bar and a 200-calorie shake that my nutrition team created to overcome the lack of good options. They are the bars and shakes that I personally use and recommend to all my clients.** Not only do they taste *delicious* but they are the perfect on the go meal combination. You can find the 3-Hour Diet™ bars and shakes online at 3hourdiet.net and nationwide anywhere bars and shakes are sold.

Option 1: Bar and Yogurt Combination

Pick one bar from list A and then one yogurt from list B.

List A (Bars)

BALANCE Bar® Cookie Dough

BALANCE Bar® Peanut Butter

BALANCE Bar® Almond Brownie

BALANCE Bar® Mocha Chip

BALANCE Bar® Chocolate Raspberry Fudge

BALANCE Bar® Honey Peanut

BALANCE Bar® Chocolate

BALANCE Bar® Mocha Chip

BALANCE Bar® Yogurt Honey Peanut

BALANCE Gold® Triple Chocolate Chaos

BALANCE Gold® Caramel Nut Blast

BALANCE Gold® Chocolate Peanut Butter

BALANCE Gold® Rocky Road

Be® Powered Protein Bar—all natural chocolate raspberry

Be® Powered Protein Bar—all natural wild berry

DETOUR White Chocolate Peanut Butter

DETOUR S'mores

DETOUR Caramel Peanut

DETOUR Peanut Butter

LUNA® Bar Nutz Over Chocolate™

LUNA® Bar Lemon Zest

LUNA® Bar S'mores

LUNA® Bar Chocolate Pecan Pie

LUNA® Bar Toasted Nuts 'n Cranberry

LUNA® Bar Chocolate Peppermint Stick

LUNA® Bar Dulce de Leche

LUNA® Bar Key Lime Pie

LUNA® Bar Cherry Covered Chocolate™

LUNA® Bar Sweet Dreams™

LUNA® Bar Chai Tea

LUNA® Bar Orange Bliss™

ZonePerfect® Apple Cinnamon

ZonePerfect® Double Chocolate

ZonePerfect® Chocolate Caramel Cluster

ZonePerfect® Lemon Yogurt

ZonePerfect® Strawberry Yogurt

ZonePerfect® Chocolate Almond Raisin

ZonePerfect® Caramel Apple

ZonePerfect® Chocolate Peanut Butter

ZonePerfect® Chocolate Mint
ZonePerfect® Chocolate Raspberry

List B (Yogurt)—200-Calorie Yogurts

Yoplait® Original Banana Crème
Yoplait® Original Berry Banana
Yoplait® Original Blackberry Harvest
Yoplait® Original Blueberry Crumble
Yoplait® Original Boysenberry
Yoplait® Original Cherry Orchard
Yoplait® Original Coconut Cream Pie
Yoplait® Original French Vanilla
Yoplait® Original Harvest Peach
Yoplait® Original Key Lime Pie
Yoplait® Original Lemon Burst
Yoplait® Original Mandarin Orange
Yoplait® Original Mixed Berry
Yoplait® Original Mountain Blueberry
Yoplait® Original Orange Crème
Yoplait® Original Peach Cobbler
Yoplait® Original Piña Colada
Yoplait® Original Pineapple

Yoplait® Original Plain

Yoplait® Original Red Raspberry

Yoplait® Original Strawberry

Yoplait® Original Strawberry Banana

Yoplait® Original Strawberry Cheesecake

Yoplait® Original Strawberry Kiwi

Yoplait® Original Strawberry Mango

Yoplait® Original Tropical Peach

Yoplait® Original White Chocolate Raspberry

Be® Seven Fruit

Be® Strawberry Banana

Dannon® Light 'n Fit™ Smoothie Strawberry Banana

Dannon® Light 'n Fit™ Smoothie Tropical

OPTION 2: Bar and Shake Combination

List A—200-Calorie Bars

3-Hour Diet™ Bar—Double Chocolate Almond

3-Hour Diet™ Bar—Fruit & Nut Crunch

3-Hour Diet™ Bar—Chocolate Caramel Crunch

3-Hour Diet™ Bar—Chocolate & Peanut Butter Fudge

List B—200 Calorie Shakes

3-Hour Diet™ Shake—Cappuccino & Crème

3-Hour Diet™ Shake—Strawberries & Crème

3-Hour Diet™ Shake—Delicious Vanilla

3-Hour Diet™ Shake—Creamy Chocolate

Visit 3hourdiet.net for new updates on approved bar options for the 3-Hour Diet™

Breakfast:
<u>Home Delivery</u> Meal Options

In my ongoing search for the finest meals and food products for myself, my family, and my on-line clients, I have created the 3-Hour Diet™ At Home fresh food delivery program. Imagine this: each week, delivered to your front door are all the fresh, most delicious, and balanced meals, snacks, and treats you need to lose weight on the 3-Hour Diet™. There is nothing for you to get from the supermarket. No shopping. All you do is eat. To learn more about the 3-Hour Diet™ At Home fresh food delivery program, go to **3hourdietathome.com**. Below are just a few samples of breakfast meal choices for this delicious program.

- Sweet potato flapjacks and eggs.
- Sweet apple crepe with scrambled egg substitute, yogurt, wheat bread, and margarine.
- Farmer's frittata with turkey ham and orange.

- Wild berry crepe with pear, wheat bread, and margarine.
- Breakfast skillet (scrambled eggs with turkey ham, new potatoes and sweet potatoes) and pineapple.
- Apple-buckwheat pancakes with ricotta and turkey ham.
- Grilled cinnamon french toast with raspberry syrup and turkey sausage.

THREE
LUNCH/DINNER ON THE GO
ALL ARE APPROXIMATELY 400 CALORIES.

Lunch/Dinner Overview

Lunch/Dinner:
<u>Fast Food</u> Meal Options

These selections are the healthiest options that fulfill the criteria of the 3-Hour Plate™.

Ordering Tips

- Order all sauces and dressings "on the side."
- Don't order anything fried; stick to entrees that include words like "grilled" or "fire-roasted," not breaded or deep-fried.
- NEVER super-size it.
- Order bottled water, iced tea, or diet soda instead of regular soda.

Baja Fresh® 1 Original "Baja Style" Taco (chicken, steak, or shrimp)

- Add Side Salad with squeeze of lime or lemon instead of dressing.

Baja Fresh® 1 Fish Taco with charbroiled fish

- Add Side Salad with squeeze of lime or lemon instead of dressing.

Boston Market® ¼ Dark Sweet Garlic Rotisserie Chicken, No Skin

- Add side of Garlic Dill New Potatoes and a side of Fruit Salad.

Boston Market® Hand-Carved Honey Glazed Ham

- Add side of Green Beans OR Green Bean Casserole and a side of Garlic Dill New Potatoes.

Burger King® Hamburger

- Add Side Garden Salad with fat-free or low-fat dressing or squeeze of lemon.

Burger King® Fire-Grilled Garden Salad with chicken or shrimp

- Add fat-free or low-fat dressing and a packet of crackers if available.

Burger King® Original WHOPPER JR.® without mayonnaise

- Add Side Garden Salad with Kraft® Fat Free Ranch Dressing.

Chick-fil-A® Chick-n-Strips® Salad

- Order with Light Italian Dressing.

Chick-fil-A® Chicken Salad Sandwich

- Order sandwich on wheat bread.
- Add Side Salad with Light Italian Dressing.

Chick-fil-A® Chargrilled Chicken Sandwich

- Order Side Salad with Reduced Fat Raspberry Vinaigrette Dressing.

Dairy Queen® BBQ Beef or Pork Sandwich

- Add Side Salad with fat-free or low-fat dressing (is available but is limited menu item).

Dairy Queen® Grilled Chicken Salad with Fat-Free Dressing

- Add package of crackers or small roll.

Del Taco® (2) Chicken Tacos Del Carbon

- Del Taco® does not have Side Salad available on their menu, so bring one of your own or bring a piece of fruit.*

El Pollo Loco® 1 Leg and 1 Thigh of Flame-Grilled Chicken

- 1 (6-inch) corn tortilla and a corn cobette or fresh vegetables.

---

*See pages 98–103 for a list of 3-Hour Diet™–approved fruits and vegetables.

Fazoli's® Chicken & Pasta Caesar Salad

- Substitute reduced calorie Italian dressing.

In-N-Out® Burger Hamburger with Onion Protein Style

- Ask for half order of french fries. Add mustard and ketchup instead of spread on burger.

In-N-Out® Burger Hamburger with Onion

- Use mustard and ketchup instead of spread.

Jack in the Box® Chicken Fajita Pita

- Add 1 Side Salad; use lemon as dressing.

Jack in the Box® Asian Chicken Salad

- Use low-fat balsamic vinaigrette dressing and add 1 Egg Roll.

KFC® Chicken Breast without skin or breading

- Add order of green beans or 3-inch corn on the cob with order of mashed potatoes without gravy; add pat of butter.

Long John Silver's™ Chicken Sandwich

- Choose any diet soda from the menu.

Long John Silver's™ Shrimp and Seafood Salad with Croutons and Crumblies®

- Choose any diet soda from the menu.

Long John Silver's™ Clam Chowder bowl

- Add 2 Corn Cobettes. Choose any diet soda from the menu.

McDonald's® Cheeseburger

- Add Side Salad with Newman's Own® Low-Fat Balsamic Vinaigrette.

McDonald's® Bacon Ranch Salad (without chicken)

- Add a Fruit n' Yogurt Parfait with or without granola for dessert.

McDonald's® Chicken McGrill®

- Add a Side Salad; use lemon as dressing or Newman's Own® Low Fat Balsamic Vinaigrette (use only half the packet).

Panda Express Sweet and Sour Chicken (single serving)

- Add serving of Mixed Vegetables from the menu.

Papa John's ® Any 1 slice of Original Crust or Thin Crust Large pizza

- Make sure your toppings are limited to one meat option (if any) and any veggies you want.

- Papa John's® does not have a salad on their menu, so make sure to get a salad or a side of veggies into your meal.

Pizza Hut® Lower Fat Pizza (12" or 14"), 2 slices

- Make sure your toppings are limited to one meat option (if any) and any veggies you want.
- Add Garden Salad with nonfat dressing or squeeze of lemon for a zesty flavor.

Pizza Hut® 12" Medium Hand-Tossed Style Pizza (1 slice)

- Make sure your toppings are limited to one meat option (if any) and any veggies you want.
- Add Garden Salad with nonfat dressing or a squeeze of lemon for a zesty flavor.

Pizza Hut® Garden Salad and 4 Buffalo Wings

- Add nonfat dressing or a squeeze of lemon to your salad for a zesty flavor.

Pizza Hut® Buffalo Wings (2 pieces)

- Add one breadstick and Garden Salad with nonfat dressing or a squeeze of lemon for a zesty flavor.

Rubio's™ Fresh Mexican Grill Pork Carnitas Street Burrito℠

- Rubio's™ does not have side salad available on their menu, so either bring one of your own or bring a piece of fruit* to complete the meal.

Rubio's™ Fresh Mexican Grill White Meat Chicken Street Burrito℠

- Rubio's™ does not have side salad available on their menu, so either bring one of your own or bring a piece of fruit* to complete the meal.

---

*See pages 98–103 for a list of 3-Hour Diet™–approved fruits and vegetables.

Rubio's™ Fresh Mexican Grill Carne Asada Steak Street Burrito℠

- Rubio's™ does not have side salad available on their menu, so either bring one of your own or bring a piece of fruit* to complete the meal.

Rubio's™ Fresh Mexican Grill Baja Grill Chicken Burrito℠

- Have only half of the burrito. Save the other half for later or split with a friend.
- Rubio's™ does not have side salad available on their menu, so either bring one of your own or bring a piece of fruit* to complete the meal.

---

*See pages 98–103 for a list of 3-Hour Diet™–approved fruits and vegetables.

Rubio's™ Fresh Mexican Grill Baja Gourmet Seafood Burrito, Shrimp (no chips or rice)

- Have only half of the burrito. Save the other half for later or split with a friend.
- Rubio's™ does not have side salad available on their menu, so either bring one of your own or bring a piece of fruit* to complete the meal.

Rubio's™ Fresh Mexican Grill Chicken Taquitos (3)

- Rubio's™ does not have side salad available on their menu, so either bring one of your own or bring a piece of fruit* to complete the meal.

Rubio's™ Fresh Mexican Grill HealthMex® Chicken Salad

- Ask for cheese to be added.

---

*See pages 98–103 for a list of 3-Hour Diet™-approved fruits and vegetables.

Sonic Grilled Chicken Sandwich

Sonic Grilled Chicken Wrap without Ranch Dressing

Subway® 6" Ham, without mayo. Salt, pepper, and mustard optional

- Add Veggie Delite® Salad with choice of lemon squeeze or Kraft® Fat Free Italian dressing, or order of soup. Choose from the following: Roasted Chicken Noodle or Minestrone.

Subway® 6" Savory Turkey Breast, without mayo. Salt, pepper, and mustard optional

- Add Veggie Delite® Salad with choice of lemon squeeze or Kraft® Fat Free Italian Dressing, or order of soup. Choose from the following: Roasted Chicken Noodle or Minestrone.

Subway® 6" Tuna Sandwich, open-faced. Salt, pepper, and mustard optional

- Add Veggie Delite® Salad with squeeze of lemon or Kraft® Fat Free Italian Dressing.

TACO BELL® Ranchero Chicken Soft Tacos "Fresco Style"

- TACO BELL® does not have a side salad available on their menu, so either bring one of your own or bring a piece of fruit* to complete the meal.

TACO BELL® Beef, Chicken, or Steak Enchirito® "Fresco Style"

- TACO BELL® does not have a side salad available on their menu, so either bring one of your own or bring a piece of fruit* to complete the meal.

* See pages 98–103 for a list of 3-Hour Diet™–approved fruits and vegetables.

TACO BELL® Beef, Chicken, or Steak Gordita Baja® "Fresco Style"

- TACO BELL® does not have a side salad available on their menu, so either bring one of your own or bring a piece of fruit* to complete the meal.

TACO BELL® (2) Grilled Steak Tacos "Fresco Style"

- TACO BELL® does not have a side salad available on their menu, so either bring one of your own or bring a piece of fruit* to complete the meal.

Wendy's® Jr. Hamburger

- Add a Side Salad with Fat Free French Salad Dressing.

---

*See pages 98–103 for a list of 3-Hour Diet™–approved fruits and vegetables.

Wendy's® Mandarin Chicken® Salad

- Add Low Fat Honey Mustard Salad Dressing.

Wendy's® Grilled Chicken Sandwich

- Add Caesar Side Salad with a squeeze of lemon in place of the dressing provided.

Wendy's® Taco Supremo Salad

- Order without sour cream and without chips.

Lunch/Dinner:
<u>Restaurant</u> Meal Options

When you go to a restaurant, it can be intimidating to ask for a meal your way—but remember, you're paying the money to be there! The establishment and servers are there to make your dining experience the best it can be, and they will be the first to assert that the customer is always right. Here are a few tips I find helpful when eating out.

- Ask for a "to-go" box before your food is even delivered. Once your plate arrives, divide food into 3-Hour Plate™ portions and put the rest in the box to eat for another meal. That way the decision is already made and you won't accidentally overindulge.

- Request all sauces and dressings on the side.

- Always request low-fat, nonfat or low-calorie salad dressings. If that's not an option, try requesting some olive oil and vinegar or lemon so you can manage the amount you use.

- Ask about preparation—select options that are grilled or baked, not fried.

- Request that bread be removed from the table once you take a piece so you're not tempted to keep nibbling and fill up before your meal arrives.

- Order "à la carte"—you don't need the whole plate of enchiladas, plus salad, chips and rice and beans. Select individual items from the "à la carte" section to keep your meal the right size.

My team and I have discovered great dining options at some nationwide chains. Although some of the meals fall into the 3-Hour Plate™, others require you to follow some of the rules above.

Applebee's® Grilled Tilapia with Mango Salsa

Applebee's® Mesquite Chicken Salad

Applebee's® Tango Chicken Sandwich

Denny's® Turkey Breast Salad

- Order with no dressing.
- Ask for dinner roll.

Denny's® Grilled Chicken Breast Salad

- Ask for dinner roll.

Godfather's Pizza™ Cheese Pizza Golden or Thin Crust, 1 slice

- Add side salad with nonfat dressing.

Godfather's Pizza™ Hawaiian Pizza, Golden or Thin Crust, 1 slice

- Add side salad with nonfat dressing.

Godfather's Pizza™ Pepperoni Pizza, Golden or Thin Crust, 1 slice

- Add side salad with nonfat dressing.

Godfather's Pizza™ Super Hawaiian Pizza, Golden or Thin Crust, 1 slice

- Add side salad with nonfat dressing.

Godfather's Pizza™ Veggie Pizza, Golden or Thin Crust, 1 slice

- Add side salad with nonfat dressing.

Mimi's Café® Half Fresh Roasted Turkey Breast Sandwich, Low Fat Menu

- Order sandwich dry (no mayo).
- Fresh fruit* as the side order.

Olive Garden Capellini Pomodoro (lunch portion)

- Add grilled chicken.
- Ask for a "to-go" box to come out with your meal and put half the chicken and pasta in the box for a meal tomorrow!

---

*See pages 98–103 for a list of 3-Hour Diet™–approved fruits and vegetables.

- Include salad with Low Fat Italian or Low Fat Parmesan Peppercorn dressing on the side.

Olive Garden Chicken Giardino (lunch portion)

Olive Garden Linguine Alla Marinara (lunch portion)

- Add grilled chicken.
- Ask for "to-go" box to come out with your meal and put half the chicken and pasta in the box for a meal tomorrow!
- Include salad with Low Fat Italian or Low Fat Parmesan Peppercorn dressing on the side.

Olive Garden Shrimp Primavera (dinner portion)

- Add grilled chicken.
- Ask for "to-go" box to come out with your meal and put half the shrimp and pasta in the box for a meal tomorrow!

Olive Garden Chicken Giardino (dinner portion)

- Ask for "to-go" box to come out with your meal and put half the chicken and pasta in the box for a meal tomorrow!
- Include salad with Low Fat Italian or Low Fat Parmesan Peppercorn dressing on the side.

Olive Garden Linguine Alla Marinara (dinner portion)

- Add grilled chicken.
- Ask for "to-go" box to come out with your meal and put half the chicken and pasta in the box for a meal tomorrow!
- Include salad with a squeeze of lemon.

P.F. Chang's China Bistro℠ Shrimp Dumpling Appetizer

- Order them steamed.

P.F. Chang's China Bistro℠ Mango Chicken

- Split this with a friend or take half home with you.

P.F. Chang's China Bistro℠ Singapore Street Noodles

- Split this with a friend or take half home with you.

Red Lobster Tilapia (lunch portion)

- Baked Potato (no topping) or Wild Rice Pilaf.
- Garden Salad with nonfat dressing.

Sbarro® Traditional Pizza; Fresh Tomato and Basil, 1 slice

- Add Mixed Garden Salad with nonfat dressing.

Souplantation®

Eating at buffets can be confusing, but if you keep the 3-Hour Plate™ portions in mind, you'll be fine. Stick to soup and salad if you want to play it safe. If they have a fresh-cut sandwich section, ask for half a salad to go with your sandwich and finish off with a vegetable soup. Or have a big salad full of yummy freebies* and nonfat dressing with your sandwich. Here are a few complete meal ideas for you:

Option 1

1 cup Classic Greek (vegetarian) Salad
1 cup Big Chunk Chicken Noodle (low-fat) Soup
Salad covered in freebies* and nonfat dressing
1 chocolate chip cookie

Option 2

1 cup Wonton Chicken Happiness soup
1 cup Deep Kettle House Chili (low-fat)
Salad covered in freebies and nonfat dressing
1 cup Jell-O®

---

*For a list of freebies, please see pages 103–107.

Option 3

1 cup Big Chunk Chicken Noodle (low-fat) Soup

½ cup Nutty Waldorf Salad

Salad covered in freebies, sprinkled with Cheddar
cheese and drizzled in nonfat dressing

1½ cups Jell-O®

Lunch/Dinner:
<u>Frozen</u> Meal Options

Frozen meals always include a salad.

Remember—these are easy to pick up at the store for a quick lunch at the office, but you need to supplement them with an easy salad. You can make the salad at home, or many grocery stores and delis have salad bars where you can put together the following:

If cheese is not in your frozen meal, choose from the following selections of salads:

- Add a large romaine lettuce salad complete with ½ cup of boiled artichoke hearts, ½ cup steamed green beans, and 1 ounce of Monterey Jack cheese. Drizzle with 1 tablespoon of low-fat or nonfat dressing, or use 1 teaspoon of flaxseed oil with a squeeze of lemon.

- Add a large spinach salad with 1 ounce of feta cheese and 1 cup steamed and sliced eggplant. Drizzle with 1 tablespoon of low-fat or nonfat balsamic dressing, or 1 teaspoon of flaxseed oil with a squeeze of lemon.

If your frozen meal does include cheese, choose from the following selections of salads:

- Add a large iceberg lettuce salad with 1 medium tomato (sliced or cubed) and 1 cup of an assortment of sliced bell peppers. Drizzle with 1 tablespoon of low-fat or nonfat dressing or use 1 teaspoon of flaxseed oil with a squeeze of lemon.

- Add a large spinach salad with whole or sliced mushrooms and a sprinkle of radish slices. Drizzle with 1 tablespoon of low-fat or nonfat balsamic dressing or 1 teaspoon of flaxseed oil with a squeeze of lemon.

Lean Cuisine®

Lean Cuisine® One Dish Favorites™ Swedish Meatballs with Pasta

Lean Cuisine® Cafe Classics Roasted Garlic Chicken

Lean Cuisine® Cafe Classics Honey Dijon Grilled Chicken

Lean Cuisine® Cafe Classics Three Cheese Chicken

Lean Cuisine® Comfort Classics Baked Chicken Florentine

Lean Cuisine® One Dish Favorites™ Chicken Chow Mein

Lean Cuisine® Comfort Classics Salisbury Steak

Lean Cuisine® Comfort Classics Meatloaf and Whipped Potatoes

Lean Cuisine® Cafe Classics Chicken with Basil Cream Sauce

Lean Cuisine® Spa Cuisine™ Classics Chicken in Peanut Sauce

Lean Cuisine® Cafe Classics Chicken Carbonara

Lean Cuisine® Comfort Classics Oven Roasted Beef

Lean Cuisine® Comfort Classics Cheese Lasagna with Chicken Scaloppini

Lean Cuisine® Cafe Classics Chicken Marsala

Lean Cuisine® Cafe Classics Chicken à l'Orange

Lean Cuisine® One Dish Favorites™ Classic Five Cheese Lasagna

Lean Cuisine® Dinnertime Selections Salisbury Steak

Lean Cuisine® Comfort Classics Beef Peppercorn

Healthy Choice®

Healthy Choice® Flavor Adventures Roasted Chicken Chardonnay

Healthy Choice® Flavor Adventures Oriental Style Beef

Healthy Choice® Flavor Adventures Grilled Chicken Caesar

Healthy Choice® Flavor Adventures Grilled Basil Chicken

Healthy Choice® Flavor Adventures Beef Merlot

Healthy Choice® Familiar Favorites Tuna Casserole

Healthy Choice® Familiar Favorites Grilled Chicken Breast & Pasta

Healthy Choice® Familiar Favorites Grilled Chicken & Mashed Potatoes

Healthy Choice® Salisbury Steak & Redskin Mashed Potatoes

Healthy Choice® Familiar Favorites Slow Roasted Turkey Breast & Mashed Potatoes

Healthy Choice® Familiar Favorites Chicken Breast and Vegetables

Healthy Choice® Familiar Favorites Chicken Fettuccini Alfredo

Healthy Choice® Familiar Favorites Country Glazed
Chicken

Healthy Choice® Familiar Favorites Oriental Style Chicken

Healthy Choice® Beef Tips Portobello

Healthy Choice® Grilled Turkey Breast

Healthy Choice® Roasted Chicken Breast

Healthy Choice® Familiar Favorites Rigatoni with
Broccoli and Chicken

Healthy Choice® Familiar Favorites Chicken Carbonara

Healthy Choice® Oven Roasted Beef

Healthy Choice® Meatloaf

Healthy Choice® Familiar Favorites Cheesy Rice and
Chicken

Healthy Choice® Familiar Favorites Mandarin Chicken

Healthy Choice® Mixed Grills Chicken with Roasted Red
Pepper Dipping Sauce

WeightWatchers® Smart Ones®

WeightWatchers® Smart Ones® Ham & Cheddar
Smartwich™ (1)

WeightWatchers® Smart Ones® Deluxe Pizza (1)

WeightWatchers® Smart Ones® Bistro Selections™
Chicken Fettuccini

WeightWatchers® Smart Ones® Bistro Selections™
Basil Chicken

WeightWatchers® Smart Ones® Bistro Selections™
Chicken Tenderloins with Barbecue Sauce

WeightWatchers® Smart Ones® Bistro Selections™
Fajita Chicken Supreme

WeightWatchers® Smart Ones® Creamy Rigatoni with
Broccoli & Chicken

WeightWatchers® Smart Ones® Fiesta Chicken

WeightWatchers® Smart Ones® Lasagna Florentine

WeightWatchers® Smart Ones® Swedish Meatballs

WeightWatchers® Smart Ones® Traditional Lasagna
with Meat Sauce

WeightWatchers® Smart Ones® Tuna Noodle Gratin

WeightWatchers® Smart Ones® Garden Veggies &
Mozzarella Smartwich™

Amy's Kitchen®

Amy's® Spinach Feta in a Pocket Sandwich

Amy's® Stuffed Pasta Shells Bowl

Amy's® Cheese Enchilada

Amy's® Vegetable Lasagna

Amy's® Santa Fe Enchilada Bowl

Amy's® Tofu Vegetable Lasagna

Amy's® Pasta Primavera

Amy's® Spinach Pizza in a Pocket Sandwich

Amy's® Cheese Pizza in a Pocket Sandwich

Amy's® Cheese Pizza Toaster Pops (2)

The Budget Gourmet®

The Budget Gourmet® Light & Healthy Beef Sirloin
Salisbury Steak

The Budget Gourmet® Light French Recipe Chicken

Michelina's®

Michelina's® Lean Gourmet Beef Stroganoff

Michelina's® Lean Gourmet Cheese Stuffed Rigatoni

Michelina's® Lean Gourmet Chicken Alfredo Florentine

Michelina's® Lean Gourmet Layered Lasagna with Meat
Sauce

Michelina's® Lean Gourmet Shrimp with Pasta and
Vegetables

Michelina's® Lean Gourmet Swedish Meatballs

Lunch/Dinner:
Bars/Shakes Meal Options

The following are the easiest lunch/dinner options for when you truly have no time. There are two options. Option 1 combines a 200-calorie bar with a 200-calorie yogurt from well-known brands. Although they do not precisely fit the nutritional requirements of the 3-Hour Diet™, when combined they get the job done. **Option 2 combines a 200-calorie bar and a 200-calorie shake that my nutrition team created to overcome the lack of good options. They are the bars and shakes that I personally use and recommend to all my clients.** Not only do they taste *delicious* but they are the perfect on the go meal combination. You can find the 3-Hour Diet™ bars and shakes at the 3hourdiet.net and nationwide anywhere bars and shakes are sold.

OPTION 1: Bar and Yogurt Combination

Pick one bar from list A and one yogurt from list B.

List A (Bars)

BALANCE Bar® Cookie Dough

BALANCE Bar® Peanut Butter

BALANCE Bar® Almond Brownie

BALANCE Bar® Chocolate Raspberry Fudge

BALANCE Bar® Honey Peanut

BALANCE Bar® Chocolate

BALANCE Bar® Mocha Chip

BALANCE Bar® Yogurt Honey Peanut

BALANCE Gold® Triple Chocolate Chaos

BALANCE Gold® Caramel Nut Blast

BALANCE Gold® Chocolate Peanut Butter

BALANCE Gold® Rocky Road

Be® Powered Protein Bar—all natural chocolate
    raspberry

Be® Powered Protein Bar—all natural wild berry

DETOUR White Chocolate Peanut Butter

DETOUR S'mores

DETOUR Caramel Peanut

DETOUR Peanut Butter
LUNA® Bar Nutz Over Chocolate™
LUNA® Bar Lemon Zest
LUNA® Bar S'mores
LUNA® Bar Chocolate Pecan Pie
LUNA® Bar Toasted Nuts 'n Cranberry

List B (Yogurt)—200-Calorie Yogurts

Yoplait® Original Banana Crème
Yoplait® Original Berry Banana
Yoplait® Original Blackberry Harvest
Yoplait® Original Blueberry Crumble
Yoplait® Original Boysenberry
Yoplait® Original Cherry Orchard
Yoplait® Original Coconut Cream Pie
Yoplait® Original French Vanilla
Yoplait® Original Harvest Peach
Yoplait® Original Key Lime Pie
Yoplait® Original Lemon Burst
Yoplait® Original Mandarin Orange
Yoplait® Original Mixed Berry
Yoplait® Original Mountain Blueberry
Yoplait® Original Orange Crème

Yoplait® Original Peach Cobbler

Yoplait® Original Piña Colada

Yoplait® Original Pineapple

Yoplait® Original Plain

Yoplait® Original Red Raspberry

Yoplait® Original Strawberry

Yoplait® Original Strawberry Banana

Yoplait® Original Strawberry Cheesecake

Yoplait® Original Strawberry Kiwi

Yoplait® Original Strawberry Mango

Yoplait® Original Tropical Peach

Yoplait® Original White Chocolate Raspberry

Be® Seven Fruit

Be® Strawberry Banana

OPTION 2: Bar and Fruit Combination

List A—200-Calorie Bars

3-Hour Diet™ Bar—Double Chocolate Almond

3-Hour Diet™ Bar—Fruit & Nut Crunch

3-Hour Diet™ Bar—Chocolate Caramel Crunch

3-Hour Diet™ Bar—Chocolate & Peanut Butter Fudge

List B—200 Calorie Shakes

3-Hour Diet™ Shake—Cappuccino & Crème

3-Hour Diet™ Shake—Strawberries & Crème

3-Hour Diet™ Shake—Delicious Vanilla

3-Hour Diet™ Shake—Creamy Chocolate

Visit 3hourdiet.net for new updates on approved bar options for the 3-Hour Diet™

Lunch/Dinner:
Home Delivery Meal Options

These meals are part of my ongoing search for the finest meals and food products. Imagine each week, delivered to your front door, are all the fresh, most delicious, and balanced meals, snacks, and treats you need to lose weight on the 3-Hour Diet™. Absolutely no cooking for you to do. Just go online, click, and it arrives at your door. To learn more about the 3-Hour Diet™ At Home fresh food delivery program, go to 3hourdietathome.com. Here are just a few lunch and dinner meal choices for this program.

- Louisiana chicken with black bean salad
- Taco salad with turkey and Cheddar cheese
- Asian roast beef salad with mushrooms
- Chicken salad with raspberry vinaigrette
- Sliced beef broil with grilled vegetables
- Grilled portobello napoleon

- Spanish chicken and rice vegetable stew
- Turkey burger with sliced potatoes
- Southwestern quesadilla with turkey
- Chicken florentine (chicken and spinach with spinach lasagna noodles)
- Roasted lamb rosemary with barley salad and sweet potatoes
- Rock lobster tail with cranberry-rice salad and roasted Sicilian vegetables
- Healthy sloppy joe hoagie
- Braised beef with roasted red potatoes
- Italian baked chicken breast with red potatoes and peas
- Grilled rainbow trout, wild rice salad and corn cobette with wheat roll

FOUR

SNACKS
ON THE GO
ALL ARE APPROXIMATELY 100 CALORIES.

Add more snacks to your day if you are over 200 pounds. See page 10 for more info.

For each specified amount, fill in the snack line on your 3-Hour Timeline™. In general, your snacks should be about 100 calories each.

I have broken down the snack list into categories:

FRESH—these snacks include fruits, vegetables, and other fun fresh snacks. Remember, it's best to have fruit for your morning snack.

SWEET TOOTH—for all you chocolate lovers, here are

some great 100-calorie snacks to satisfy that sweet
tooth in us all.

CRUNCHY-SALTY—it's always great to have a handful
of pretzels or even potato chips.

NABISCO SNACK PACKS—for those of us really on the
go, just grab these pre-packaged snacks from
Nabisco, crack open and enjoy.

COFFEE Houses—for those of you who need a pick-
me-up during the day, we have listed some great
snack-size beverages and treats. Remember, if your
drink is caffeinated you need to drink an extra glass
of water that day!

Fresh

Apple, green or red (1 medium)

Apple juice (1 cup)

Applesauce, unsweetened (1 cup)

Apricots (8)

Bananas (1)

Bell pepper, green, yellow, red (1)

Bitter Melon—1

Blackberries (1½ cups)

Blueberries (1½ cups)

Boysenberries (1½ cups)

Broccoli (2 cups)

Cantaloupe (2 cups cubes)

Casaba Melon (2 cup cubes)

Carrots (2 cups)

Cauliflower (2 cups)

Celery and Peanut Butter (3 sticks with 1 teaspoon peanut butter on each)

Cherries (24 large)

Clementine (2)

Craisins® (4 tablespoons)

Cranberries, unsweetened (2 cups)

Cranberry juice (1 cup)

Dannon® DanActive® (any flavor)

Dannon® Light 'n Fit™ Smoothie, all flavors (1 bottle)

Dannon® Light 'n Fit Yogurt with Fiber, all flavors (6 ounces)

Dannon® Light 'n Fit™ Creamy, all flavors (6 ounces)

Dates (6)

Earthbound Farm® Organic Carrot Dippers with Organic Ranch Dip (1)

Figs, dried (2)

Figs, fresh (4)

Fruit cocktail (1 cup)

Grapefruit (1)

Grapefruit juice (1 cup)

Grapes, green or red (24)

Guava (3 small)

Honeydew (2 cups cubes)

Jell-O® Brand Smoothie Snacks (any flavor)

Kiwifruit (2 large)

Knudsen® On the Go! low-fat cottage cheese (1)

Mandarin orange segments (1½ cups)

Mango (1 medium)

McDonald's® Minute Maid® Apple Juice Box (1)

Motts® Applesauce—Cinnamon or Strawberry (1 snack size)

Nectarine (2 medium)

Orange (2 medium)

Orange Juice (1 cup)

Papaya (2 cups cubes)

Snow Peas (2 cups)

Peach (2 medium)

Pear, green (2 small)

Pepino melon (2 cups cubes)

Persimmon (4)

Pickles (4 large)

Pineapple, canned, packed in juice (⅔ cup)

Pineapple juice (1 cup)

Plum (3 medium)

Pomegranate (Chinese Apple) (1 medium)

Prickly pear (2 medium)

Prunes/dried plums (3)

Prune juice (⅔ cup)

Raisins 30

Rhubarb, sweetened (1 cup)

Raspberries (1½ cups)

Strawberries (2 cups)

Tangerine (4 small)

Vegetable juice, low-sodium (2 cups)

Watermelon (2 cups cubes)

Sweet Tooth

3-Hour Diet™ Snack Bar—Chocolate Chip

3-Hour Diet™ Snack Bar—Crunchy Oat & Almond

Angel food cake (2-ounce slice)

Baker's® cookie (www.bbcookies.com) (1)

Brownie (1 small)

Butterscotch (4 pieces)

Candy corn (20 pieces)

Chocolate-covered almonds (7)

Fudge (1 ounce)

Gelatin (½ cup)

Graham crackers, 2½-inch squares (3)

Granola bar, low-fat (1)

Gumdrops (1 ounce)

Healthy Choice®: Fudge Bar (1)

Healthy Choice®: Strawberry and Cream Bar (1)

Heath® toffee bar (1 snack size)

Hershey's® Bites Reese's® Peanut Butter (7)

Hershey's® Bites Heath® Toffee (7)

Hershey's® Bites Kit Kat® Wafers (8)

Hershey's® Bites Mini Rolo® Caramels (9)

Hershey's® Bites mr. Goodbar® Chocolate (11)

Hershey's® Bites York® Peppermint Pattie (9)

Hershey's® Bites White Chocolate Pretzels (11)

Hershey's® Kisses (4)

Hershey's® Kit Kat® (1 2-piece bar)

Hershey's® Miniatures Bar, any flavor (2)

Hershey's® Miniatures Nut Lovers, any flavor (2)

Hershey's® Sweet Escapes (1 bar, any kind)

Kellogg's® Cocoa Krispies® Cereal & Milk Bar (1)

Kellogg's® Tony's Cinnamon Krunchers Cereal & Milk
   Bar (1)

Kudos® Milk Chocolate Granola Bar with M&M's (1)

McDonald's® Apple Dippers with Low Fat Caramel Dip

M&M's® Milk Chocolate (1 mini bag)

M&M's® Peanut, fun size (1 bag)

M&M's® Peanut Butter, fun size (1 bag)

Milky Way® Dark, Fun Size (1)

Nature Valley® Granola Bar, all flavors (1 bar)

No Pudge! Fat Free Fudge Brownie
   (www.nopudge.com) (1 2-inch square)

PayDay®, snack size (1)

Peanut brittle (1 ounce)

Popsicle® Creamsicle® Bar (1)

Popsicle® Fudgsicle® Bar (1)

Pound cake (1-ounce slice)

Power Bar® Pria® Bar, all flavors (1 bar)

Pudding cup, fat-free (1)

Reese's® Peanut Butter Cup (1 snack size)

See's® Lollipop, any flavor (1)

Sherbet (½ cup)

Stretch Island Fruit Leather, any flavor (2)

The Skinny Cow® Fat Free Fudge bar (1)

The Skinny Cow® Low Fat Ice Cream Sandwich (½)

Tofutti Brand® nondairy frozen dessert, any flavor (¼ cup)

Whoppers® malted milk balls (9)

Yogurt, frozen, low-fat or nonfat (½ cup)

Yogurt, low-fat or nonfat (6 ounces)

Crunchy/Salty

Almonds (12)

Baked! Cheetos Snacks® Crunchy (1 small bag)

Breadsticks, 4-inch long (2)

Cashews (12)

Chips, baked, tortilla or potato (¾ ounce or 15–20 chips)

GeniSoy® Soy Crisps (25)

Handi-Snacks® Mister Salty® Pretzels 'n Cheez (1 pack)

Jolly Time Minis Healthy Pop Butter Flavor (1 bag)

Melba toast (4 slices)

Nabisco® Ritz Chip®, Cheddar (10 chips)

Nabisco® Ritz Chip®, Original (10 chips)

Nabisco® Ritz Chip®, Sour Cream & Onion (10 chips)

Orville Redenbacher's® Popcorn Mini Cakes, all flavors
(10 cakes)

Oyster crackers (24)

Peanuts (20)

Pecans (8 halves)

Pepperidge Farm® Goldfish® Crisps, Four Cheese (25)

Popcorn, air-popped (3 cups)

Potato chips, fat-free (15–20)

Pretzels (¾ ounce)

Pringles® Reduced Fat Original, Snack Stack® (1 pack)

Pumpkin seeds (⅓ cup)

Quaker® Quakes Corn Rings, Cheddar Cheese (20)

Quaker® Quakes Corn Rings, Nacho Cheese (20)

Quaker® Quakes Corn Rings, BBQ (20)

Rice cakes (2)

Saltine crackers (6)

Sargento®, Cheese Dip & Sticks (1 pack)

Sesame seeds (2 tablespoons)

Soda crackers (4)

String cheese (1)

Sunflower seeds (2 tablespoons)

Sunshine® Cheez-It® Twisterz™ (12)

Tortilla chips, fat-free (15–20)
Trader Joe's Low Fat Rice Crisps, Caramel (14 crisps)
Trader Joe's Low Fat White Cheddar Corn Crisps (20 crisps)
Uncle Sam Cereal (½ cup dry)
Whole wheat crackers (2–5)

Snack Packs

Nabisco® 100 Calorie Pack, Chips Ahoy!® Thin Crisps (1 bag)
Nabisco® 100 Calorie Pack, Fruit Snacks® Mixed Berry (1 bag)
Nabisco® 100 Calorie Pack, Kraft® Cheese Nips® Thin crisps (1 bag)
Nabisco® 100 Calorie Pack, Oreo® thin crisps (1 bag)
Nabisco® 100 Calorie Pack, Wheat Thins® Minis (1 bag)
Nabisco® 100 Calorie Pack, Honey Maid® Cinnamon Thin Crisps (1 bag)
Nabisco® 100 Calorie Pack, Ritz® Snack Mix (1 bag)

Coffee House

Starbucks® Beverages

Grande Nonfat Cappuccino

Grande Nonfat Caffè Latte
Tall Nonfat Sugar-free Vanilla Latte
Tall Nonfat Sugar-free Iced Vanilla Latte
Grande Iced Shaken Coffee
Grande Tazo® Shaken Iced Tea (black or Passion™)
Tall Tazo® Tea Lemonade

Starbucks® Snacks

Starbucks has some great snacks that you can enjoy with a regular coffee, complete with non-fat milk and Splenda®. Remember to have only one of these snacks.

Chocolate Hazelnut Biscotti
Vanilla Almond Biscotti
Madeleine

The Coffee Bean & Tea Leaf®

Nonfat Cappuccino, Single
Nonfat Cafe Latte, 12 ounces
Iced Cappuccino with whole milk, 16 ounces
Nonfat Iced Cappuccino, 24 ounces
Iced Cafe Latte with whole milk, 16 ounces
Nonfat Iced Cafe Latte, 24 ounces

Iced Mocha Latte with Fat Free No Sugar Added
Powder, 16 ounces

Iced Vanilla Latte with Fat Free No Sugar Added
Powder, 16 ounces

Iced Chai Tea Latte with Fat Free No Sugar Added
Powder, 24 ounces

Cafe Vanilla with Fat Free No Sugar Added Powder, 12
ounces

Cafe Mocha with Fat Free No Sugar Added Powder, 12
ounces

Chai Ice Blended® with Fat Free No Sugar Added
Powder, 12 ounces

eXtreme Ice Blended® with Fat Free No Sugar Added
Powder, 12 ounces

"Gas Station Gourmet"

We've all been there—you're stuck on the
road and it's time for your next snack. This section includes a list of food items commonly
found at most gas station mini-marts. Use this
list to help you make smart selections when
you're car-bound.

Fruit cocktail (1 cup)

Grapefruit juice (1 cup)

Jell-O® Brand Smoothie Snacks (any flavor)

Orange Juice (1 cup)

Pineapple juice (1 cup)

Raisins (30)

Vegetable juice, low-sodium (2 cups)

Candy corn (20 pieces)

Chocolate-covered almonds (7)

Graham crackers, 2½-inch squares (3)

Granola bar, low-fat (1)

Gumdrops (1 ounce)

Hershey's® Kisses (4)

Kit Kat® (1 2-piece bar)

Nature Valley® Granola Bar, all flavors (1 bar)

Pudding cup, fat-free (1)

Whoppers® malted milk balls (9)

Almonds (12)

Baked! Cheetos® Snacks Crunchy (1 small bag)

Cashews (12)

Handi-Snacks® Mister Salty® Pretzels 'n Cheez (1 pack)

Peanuts (20)

Popcorn, air-popped (3 cups)

Potato chips, fat-free (15–20)

Pretzels (¾ ounce)

Pumpkin seeds (⅓ cup)

Rice cakes (2)

Saltine crackers (6)

String cheese (1)

Tortilla chips, fat-free (15–20)

FIVE

TREATS ON THE GO

ALL ARE APPROXIMATELY 30–50 CALORIES

Treats

For each specified amount, fill in the treat line on your 3-Hour Timeline™. Eat a delicious treat every day. In general, they should be 30 to 50 calories.

3-Hour Diet™ Daily Treat—Rich Chocolate
3 Musketeers® Miniatures (2)
Animal crackers (4)
Caramel piece (2½-ounce piece)
Cheese slice, reduced-calorie (1)

Chocolate chips (½ tablespoon)

Chocolate-coated mints (4)

Cookie, butter (1)

Cookie, fat-free (1 small)

Cookie, fortune (1)

Corn cake (1)

Crackers, Triscuit® (2)

Cranberry sauce (¼ cup)

European chestnuts (1 ounce)

Frozen seedless grapes (1 cup)

Gelatin dessert, sugar-free (1)

Gingersnaps (3)

Ginkgo nuts (1 ounce or 14 medium)

Graham crackers (1 2½-inch square)

Gumdrops (2)

Hard candy (1)

Hershey's® Bites Reese's® Peanut Butter (4)

Hershey's® Bites Heath® Toffee (4)

Hershey's® Bites Kit Kat® Wafers (4)

Hershey's® Bites Mini Rolo® Caramels (5)

Hershey's® Bites Mr. Goodbar® Chocolate (5)

Hershey's® Bites York® Peppermint Pattie (5)

Hershey's® Bites White Chocolate Pretzels (6)

Hershey's® Nuggets®, any flavor (1)

Nestlé® Signatures™ Turtles® bite size (1)

Popsicle® Mighty Magic Mini's (1)

Popsicle® Swirlwinds™ Ice Pops (1)

Popsicle® Red, White & Blue Ice Pops (1)

Popsicle® A•C•E Juice Pops (1)

Popsicle® Sugar Free Creamsicle® Pops (2)

Switzer's™ Cherry Bites (12)

Switzer's™ Black Licorice Bites (12)

Hershey's® Hugs® or Kisses (2)

Hershey's® Miniatures Bar, any flavor (1)

Hershey's® Miniatures Nut Lovers, any flavor (1)

Ice milk, vanilla (¼ cup)

Ice pop, made with water (2-ounce pop)

Jelly beans (7)

Licorice twist (1)

Life Savers®, all fruit flavors (3)

Lollipop, Life Savers®, swirled flavors (1)

M&M's® (¼ of small bag)

M&M's® Minis (¼ of tube)

Marshmallow (1 large)

Marshmallows, mini (¼ cup)

McDonald's® Kiddie Cone

Miss Meringue® cookie (www.missmeringue.com) (1)

Nestlé® Crunch® miniature (1)

Nonfat ice cream (½ cup) drizzled with Hershey® Syrup

Oreo® cookie (1)

Popcorn, air-popped (1 cup)

Pretzels (½ ounce)

Prune (1)

Raisins (1 tablespoon)

Raisins, chocolate covered (10)

Reese's® Peanut Butter Cup (1)

Rice Krispies Treats® square (½)

Ritz Bits®, peanut butter (5)

SnackWell's® sandwich cookie (1)

Starburst® Fruit Chew (3 pieces)

Stretch Island Fruit Leather, any flavor (1)

Teddy Grahams®, Honey (6)

Tootsie Roll® Pop® any flavor (1)

Vanilla wafers (2)

York® Peppermint Pattie (1 small)

Fruit List

The following fruits are acceptable and portioned to add to any of your On-the-Go meals.

However, if you are choosing to have one of the bar and fruit or shake and fruit options and need a 100-calorie fruit to complete your meal, please select any two of the items below.

Apples, green or red (1 medium)
Apple juice (½ cup)
Applesauce, unsweetened (½ cup)
Apricots (4)
Bananas (½ medium)
Blackberries (¾ cup)
Blueberries (¾ cup)
Boysenberries (¾ cup)
Cantaloupe (⅓ melon, or 1 cup cubes)
Casaba melon (⅓ melon or 1 cup cubes)
Cherries (12 large)
Clementine
Craisins® (2 tablespoons)
Cranberries, unsweetened (1 cup)
Cranberry juice (½ cup)
Dates (3)
Figs, dried (1)
Figs, fresh (2)

Fruit cocktail (½ cup)

Grapefruit (½)

Grapefruit juice (½ cup)

Grapes, green or red (12)

Guava (1½ small)

Honeydew (⅛ melon, or 1 cup cubes)

Kiwifruit (1 large)

Mandarin orange (¾ cup)

Mango (½ medium)

Nectarine (1 medium)

Orange (1 medium)

Orange juice (½ cup)

Papaya (½ medium or 1 cup)

Peach (1 medium)

Pear, green (1 small)

Pepino melon (1 cup cubes)

Persimmon (2)

Pineapple, canned, packed in juice (⅓ cup)

Pineapple juice (½ cup)

Plum (2 medium)

Pomegranate (Chinese Apple) (½ medium)

Prickly pear (1 medium)

Prunes/dried plums (2)

Prune juice (⅓ cup)
Raisins (2 tablespoons)
Rhubarb, sweetened (½ cup)
Raspberries (1 cup)
Strawberries (1 cup)
Tangerine (2 small)
Watermelon (1 cup cubes)

Vegetable List

The following vegetables are acceptable and portioned to add to any of your On-the-Go meals. However, if you are choosing to have one of our bar or shake options and need a 100-calorie serving of vegetables to complete your meal, please select any two of the items below. All servings are 2 cups raw or 1 cup cooked, unless otherwise stated.

Artichoke, medium
Artichoke hearts, boiled
Asparagus
Bean sprouts
Beet greens

Beets

Bell peppers (green, yellow, red)

Bitter melon

Broccoli

Brussels sprouts

Carrots

Cauliflower

Celeriac

Chard

Chayote (squash)

Collard greens

Eggplant

Fennel bulb

Green beans

Kale

Kohlrabi

Leeks

Mung bean sprouts

Okra

Onions (1 cup raw, ⅔ cup cooked)

Parsnips

Pea pods

Pickles (4 large)

Pimento, sweet (1 cup)

Rutabaga

Sauerkraut

Scallion

Seaweed, raw

Snow peas

Spinach

String beans

Tomatillo, raw (2 medium)

Tomato (2 medium)

Tomato paste (4 tablespoons)

Tomato puree (1 cup)

Tomato sauce (1 cup)

Tomatoes, canned (1 cup)

Turnips

Vegetable juice, low-sodium (1 cup)

Vegetable soup, fat-free, low-sodium (1 cup)

Freebies

Freebies are foods that have less than 20 calories per serving. The following items do not need to be counted and can be consumed as often as you like. These are great items to use if you want a second plate of food or more than your two daily snacks. Enjoy them!

Vegetables

Alfalfa sprouts

Cabbage

Celery

Cucumber

Green onions (scallions)

Jalapeño and other hot peppers

Jicama

Lettuce, all types (iceberg, loose-leaf, romaine, spinach, watercress)

Mushrooms

Radishes

Zucchini

Drinks

Canarino® Italian hot lemon drink (www.canarino.com)

Carbonated or mineral water (add lime or lemon for great taste!)

Coffee, plain

Soft drinks, calorie-free

Tea

Seasonings

Chef Bernard's Fennel Pollen Spice Blends™
(www.chefbernard.com)

Garlic

Ginger

Herbs, fresh or dried

Kernel Season's Gourmet Popcorn Seasoning
(www.kernelseasons.com—also excellent on pasta,
vegetables, chicken, potatoes, eggs, and pita)

Lawry's® Seasoned Salt

Lemongrass

Lemon pepper

Mrs. Dash®

Natural extracts (lemon, orange, vanilla, mint, etc.)

Nonstick olive oil cooking spray

Peppers and peppercorns (hot chili, black, white, pink,
green)

Poppy seeds

Saffron

Salt (kosher, sea salt, fleur de sel, seasoning, Morton®)

Sesame seeds, pumpkin seeds (pepitas)

Spice blends (Cajun, curry, five spice, jerk, pickling, poultry)

Star anise

Tabasco® (hot pepper sauce)

Togarashi (Japanese chili pepper)

Vanilla (whole-bean, powder, paste, natural extract)

Wasabi powder

Condiments

Cured olives

Grape seed oil

Horseradish

Lemon juice

Lemon myrtle oil

Lime juice

Mustard

Nut oils (walnut, pistachio, almond, macadamia, hazelnut)

Pepperoncinis

Pickled ginger

Pickled relish

Pickles, capers, cornichons

Salsa fresca

Truffle oil

Vinegars (balsamic, seasoned rice, sherry, naturally flavored)

Walden Farms® calorie-free salad dressings (www.waldendfarms.com)

Yuzu juice

SIX

BONUS RESOURCES

Success Stories Secrets

Anywhere Visualizations

How to Drink Alcohol

Calorie-Free Drinks

Eating at Events

n this bonus section, you will find a number of bonus resources designed to keep you inspired on your 3-Hour Diet™ journey. First, I want to share a number of success stories from my clients who took the 3-Hour challenge and won. In these stories, they share their powerful secrets to success!

HEIGHT: 5'7½"

AGE: 40

STARTING WEIGHT: 207 lbs.

CURRENT WEIGHT: 130 lbs.

OTHER: Married 17 years
with twins (a boy and a
girl); works part-time at an
elementary school

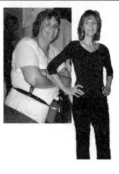

"Last August after a long vacation in Florida with
my husband and 13-year-old twins, I could no
longer look at myself in a photo let alone a mirror.
One morning I woke up to my favorite show *Good
Morning America*, and there was Jorge talking with
Diane Sawyer.

"I wanted a healthy plan because I knew from taking the dieting plunge so many times that I did not
want to deprive myself or I would quit as I always did.

"I started eating the way Jorge recommended.
Looking at my dinner plate in a whole new way

seemed too easy but I loved it! That first week I was feeling better than I had felt in years and I lost 7 pounds! On my birthday I reached my goal weight and I feel younger and better than ever."

MICHELE'S SECRETS TO SUCCESS

- Prioritize everything that is important, either in your head or on a calendar or piece of paper.

- Get ready the night before for your next day. Have lunches and dinners decided for the week so that when you go shopping you only get the things you need.

- Keep it healthy—don't deprive yourself!

HEIGHT: 5'3"

AGE: 25

STARTING WEIGHT: 131 lbs.

CURRENT WEIGHT: 118 lbs.

OTHER: Works full time (12- to 14-hour days); very little free time

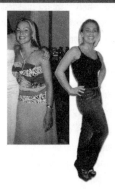

"Before Jorge Cruise, I saw a heavy, struggling, tired person. Someone who exercised but many times ate too much (and knew it), snacked too often, and craved sugar all the time. I was consistently disappointed with the way pants fit, my face in photos, my thighs in general, and the size of my calves.

"I saw my mom recently and she exclaimed, 'You look so skinny!' My mom's comment and other people's comments motivate me to further my efforts in maintaining my weight and my commitment to Jorge's great, easy, explainable 3-hour plan. Not only can I explain why the plan works to myself but I can also explain it to others—it is a livable plan."

CLAIRE'S SECRETS TO SUCCESS

- Plan! Plan! Plan!

- If you have a hectic schedule, have lots of snacks like Pria bars, almonds, fruit, and other easy-to-eat items close at hand.

- Drink a glass of water before you go out or go shopping so you're not empty when you order or arrive, and then eat the wrong thing or too much.

AGE: 40

STARTING WEIGHT: 310 lbs.

CURRENT WEIGHT: 155 lbs.

OTHER: Happily married stay-at-home mom of three children

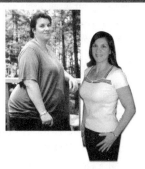

"The image in the mirror before I started Jorge Cruise's 3-Hour Diet™ was not me. I did not know who that person was. I felt I was wearing a sign for the world to see that said 'undisciplined woman who can't lose weight.' I was constantly thinking about my weight. I would tell myself, 'I need to do something,' 'tomorrow I will be good,' 'I'll never be able to lose over a hundred pounds' and so on.

"From the very first day, I knew this was different. Eating every three hours helped me to focus on what I was eating, how much I was eating, and how often I was eating. It helped me stop all the 'mindless eating' and to make better and healthier choices.

"I'm now a woman taking charge of her health and her life. I'm proud that I worked hard and sweated off every pound. When I look in the mirror now, I know the woman looking back at me!"

MARIA'S SECRETS TO SUCCESS

- Make lists. Plan ahead for the next day and just do it!

- Buy a journal to keep track of your eating and exercise routine. Mark off every day that you exercise. Once you see all of the marks, you'll be motivated to keep it up.

- Add in Jorge's 8 Minutes in the Morning® exercises for more fat burning, toning, and firming!

AGE: 38

STARTING WEIGHT: 245 lbs.

CURRENT WEIGHT: 195 lbs.

OTHER: A father of 3 small children; works as an interpreter and actor

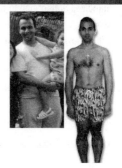

"Before the 3-Hour Diet™, I was not comfortable with my body. At first I thought it was part of getting older and being a dad. My acting career was at a standstill. I was a dad who had no energy for his kids.

"I was booked for a small role on a prime-time show (*Law & Order: SVU*). I was playing a morgue assistant and when they asked me what size scrubs they thought I wore, I told them large. I was wrong. They had to get me an XL. When I saw my brief moment on television I saw a fuller face than I was expecting.

"I started the 3-Hour Diet™ as a birthday gift to myself and have now been doing Jorge's program consistently for a year. I have become a poster child for Jorge's program in my neighborhood, at my job, and to family members. I feel motivated because I have motivated others."

DENNIS'S SECRETS TO SUCCESS

- If you have kids, aim to set a good example for them.

- Watch television programs that make you think about your health, such as those offered on Discovery Health.

- Make your morning exercises a routine, as routine as brushing your teeth. If you can, do Jorge's 8 Minute Moves™ right in the bathroom after you brush your teeth.

AGE: 44

STARTING WEIGHT:
324 lbs.

CURRENT WEIGHT:
233 lbs.

OTHER: A happily
married full-time
meteorologist and
published author.

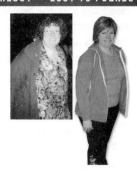

"Before I started Jorge's plan I was just *existing*. I didn't truly care for myself and was constantly doing things for others. I also had many 'thorns' to deal with, including the sudden loss of my father, caring for my chronically ill husband and constantly rotating shifts at my job.

"Everything has changed since I started the plan—not only my physical appearance, which surprises me every day, but the way I feel on the inside. I feel so much happier about myself. I'm learning about what I have going on with ME—thinking about ME first, taking care of myself first, and then letting everything else in my life fall into place.

"In addition to my weight loss and healthy outlook, my cholesterol and blood pressure have dropped. I can no longer wear plus size '1X' tops; they're way too big for me!"

ELEANOR'S SECRETS TO SUCCESS

- Communication—This is *key!!* You must keep in touch with others in order to understand yourself and to get the help and support you need to succeed!

- Do your 8 Minute Moves™ every day! Keep going, even if you don't feel up to it. You will feel better when you do.

- Journal, journal, journal! Get to know what makes you tick, and what ticks you off. Get it off your mind by writing it down. You'll feel better!

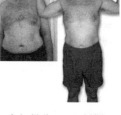

HEIGHT: 5'10"

AGE: 53

STARTING WEIGHT: 228 lbs.

CURRENT WEIGHT: 188 lbs.

OTHER: A retired naval officer working a second career in information technology; married with three grandchildren.

"Before the 3-Hour Diet™ I was ashamed that I had let myself get so out of shape! I was embarrassed at how I looked and was not comfortable in my clothes.

"I was raised thinking that I had to finish everything on my plate. Now, once I feel full, I stop eating even if there is still food left. What a relief. It didn't take me long to realize I could eat my fill, feel full, and still stay on Jorge's plan. I lost weight doing it this way and I love the results!

"Since being on Jorge's program, I am comfortable with myself, I fit into my clothes, my wife loves how I look, and I can look in the mirror at my slimmer body and feel good about how I look. I am more confident at work because I feel better about myself."

PAUL'S SECRETS TO SUCCESS

- Prioritize! Prioritize! Prioritize! Look at what you have to do for the day, week, month, and prioritize those tasks.

- Feel good about yourself. Find snacks you like and enjoy them. My favorite snacks are trail mix and yogurt cups.

- When you get the urge to eat, ask yourself whether that urge is based on true hunger or an emotional need.

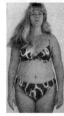

HEIGHT: 5'7½"

AGE: 33

STARTING WEIGHT: 187 lbs.

CURRENT WEIGHT: 135 lbs.

OTHER: a stay-at-home mom with 2 young children

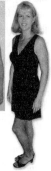

"Ten months ago, when I looked in the mirror, I saw: Mother, Wife, Daughter, Sister, Niece, Granddaughter, Aunt, Cousin . . . the list goes on and on. I put everyone and everything else first. I had a 2-month-old and a 3-year-old. I think when I decided to give everything to my kids, I lost myself.

"After my now 3-year-old son was born, I joined an expensive gym, wanting to make the effort. But of course I never went. I didn't stick with it because of the lack of financial resources and lack of willpower.

"The 3-Hour Diet™ changed my life. Sure, I lost the 52 pounds I set out to lose. But something else happened. I transformed on the inside as well. I love myself more. I love my husband and kids more (if that's possible). When I look in the mirror now, I have finally found ME behind the Mother, Wife, Daughter, and Sister."

TASHA'S SECRETS TO SUCCESS

- Keep food temptations out of the house. When it's out of sight, it's out of your mouth.

- Plan your day and your week ahead of time.

- Always have healthy snacks in your car or purse so that you can stay on schedule.

- When you go to a social setting, try to focus on the importance of the people and not the food. Eat a healthy snack ahead of time or bring a healthy option to share.

- Stay focused on why you want to lose the weight and have a healthier lifestyle.

HEIGHT: 5'3"

AGE: 56

STARTING WEIGHT:
252 lbs.

CURRENT WEIGHT:
187 lbs.

OTHER: Full-time career
woman, grandmother of 3

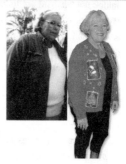

"Before I started the 3-Hour Diet™ I was pretty much okay with myself, even though I knew my weight was a problem. It didn't affect my ability to do things. I was active in sports and always had a fun social life.

"I was never that concerned; whenever I wanted to lose 40 pounds I'd eliminate carbs from my diet. I'd lose quickly, but then I'd gradually gain it back plus more. I didn't care if the diet was healthy and I yo-yo'd all my life.

"Now I get it. It's about a lifestyle change. I still

eat what I want, but I've learned the nutritional value associated with it. Instead of depriving myself of things, I eat them in moderation. The best thing is when I get off track a little (which happens), I don't gain. I don't have to go back and start over. It's the first time in my life I've kept 65 pounds off."

PHYLLIS'S SECRETS TO SUCCESS

- Put your meals in your computer scheduler so it will beep and remind you to eat.

- Know that being healthy is your choice. Do it for you.

- Create a weight-loss group at 3hourdiet.net; it's a great support network and a fun way to meet new people.

HEIGHT: 5'3"

AGE: 34

STARTING WEIGHT:
175 lbs.

CURRENT WEIGHT:
139 lbs.

OTHER: Married full-
time professional

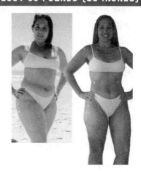

"I had tried and failed at weight loss many times. It seemed as if I was always dieting, but never making any progress. I felt frumpy. I would hide behind huge, baggy clothes and hated to shop because nothing ever fit. I fell into a sedentary lifestyle where food became my pleasure.

"It wasn't until the Jorge Cruise plan that I learned to eat balanced meals. I never realized how many calories were in some of the fast-food and junk-food choices I made on a weekly basis. Many times I would eat as many calories in one meal as I now eat in an entire day. I'm amazed that I don't crave those bad foods anymore, and that I am comfortable knowing how to make the right choices. This has definitely been an easy program to follow and I have seen amazing results. Who knew it could be this easy and enjoyable?"

KAREN'S SECRETS TO SUCCESS

- Plan breakfast time based on a certain event for the day. For example, if you have a business luncheon at noon, eat breakfast at 6 a.m., followed by a snack 3 hours later.

- Keep a freezer full of frozen entrees, so you can grab a quick meal without much preparation.

- Remember, nothing is off limits, you just have to be mindful of how much to eat and when to eat it.

CATHY ARREDONDO—LOST 70 POUNDS

HEIGHT: 5'5"

AGE: 47

STARTING WEIGHT: 235 lbs.

CURRENT WEIGHT: 165 lbs.

OTHER: A single mom with 2 grown children; works full time

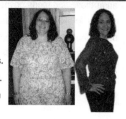

"Before the 3-Hour Diet™, I was miserable. I'd been an overweight child, an overweight teenager, and an overweight adult. My weight continued to climb through two pregnancies and a divorce. At the age of 30, I was diagnosed with lupus. My medication not only caused me to gain 50 more pounds but made my body and face look bloated. I looked like a balloon.

"I discovered the 3-Hour Diet™. Finally, a program that makes sense! The food plan seemed easy to follow. I believed this program would work and that I was worth the effort. I realized I could no longer continue to live my life this way. I had had enough!

Now, I am truly amazed at my appearance. It still surprises me! I sometimes catch a glimpse of myself in a reflection and it takes me a minute to realize 'Hey, that's me!' "

CATHY'S SECRETS TO SUCCESS

- Face your emotional issues head-on rather than using food to solve them.
- Plan and prepare meals and snacks ahead of time.
- Get support from family and friends.
- Keep a scrapbook that details your weight-loss journey.

HEIGHT: 5'4"

AGE: 45

STARTING WEIGHT: 240 lbs.

CURRENT WEIGHT: 155 lbs.

OTHER: Busy wife, mother
of three small children

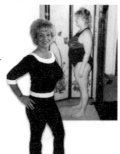

"After having my third child I looked in the mirror one
day and realized I didn't recognize myself anymore. I
had my children 18 months apart and late in my life.
Although I loved my children and my husband I found
myself very unhappy with my life. I just figured this
was motherhood and I better get used to it.

"My weight (or the way I felt at this weight) was
hurting my relationships with both my children and
my husband. This stressed me out and I ate more. I
began trying every diet I could find and would lose

weight in the first two weeks, but would put it all back on in the next few weeks."

"It wasn't until I met Jorge Cruise and started doing his 3-Hour Diet™ that I found myself losing weight and at the same time eating more food than I had eaten in the past. I began seeing the changes and then feeling the changes in me. I started looking in the mirror and caught myself smiling back. My family noticed these positive changes too. I was becoming me again. What a great feeling!

"I now wake up every morning excited and eager to get in shape, and healthier than I've ever been. I have more energy to keep up with my three kids and yes, energy left over to enjoy time with my husband.

"Life is great!"

LORI'S SECRETS TO SUCCESS

- Surround yourself with healthy choices.
- Buy an outfit in the next size down and aim to fit in it.
- Carry healthy snacks in your purse so you don't get hungry on the go and make a bad choice.

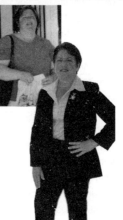

One of my most successful clients, Susan Rosenberg, is a star when it comes to grocery shopping and portioning her food. I thought it'd be great to include an update on her continued success and asked her to share some of her best tips!

Since first being featured in *The 3-Hour Diet*™ she has lost 33 more pounds for a total of 120 lost!

HEIGHT: 5'3"

AGE: 45

STARTING WEIGHT: 273 lbs.

CURRENT WEIGHT: 153 lbs.

OTHER: Mother of a 22-year-old son in college; executive with a nationwide corporation.

"In January 2004, six months before starting the 3-Hour Diet™, I became a vegetarian and gained even more weight, finally topping off at 287! I managed to lose 10 pounds by learning more about the proper way to eat vegetarian.

"I saw Jorge on the news at the end of May 2004 and applied to be part of his *3-Hour Diet* book. When I was contacted that I was selected I cried. I also realized that this was a sign of a new beginning for me. I never missed a meeting and I lived the 3-Hour Diet™ religiously.

"After a few weeks of losing 2 to 3 pounds per week I went one step further and started portioning out every meal and every snack. My motto is 'nothing stays in my house in its original package.'

"I am very busy like most people, taking care of my mother's needs at home, caring for my disabled sister and brother-in-law 100 miles away, and working for a major corporation. I also do a lot of volunteering for animal rescue every day.

"Even with all of that I know I have no excuse for failing if I plan ahead! Every Sunday I shop in the morning and prepare my weekly meals and snacks. Every other Sunday I spend time preparing soups, chili, stir-fries, and my own frozen dinners. All in all it takes most of the morning on those Sundays.

"Monday through Sunday I have gallon-size Ziplok® bags with the entire day's food inside. I never go anywhere without my personal cooler and my water. I always carry extra meal bars just in case. I eat a lot of fresh fruit and veggies for my snacks as I feel they are much more satisfying. I also always wear my 3-hour timer—even now I might miss my eating time if I don't pay attention.

"I never let anything get in the way and I am able to keep my schedule as well as everyone else's as I am always prepared. No matter what, I never leave home without my cooler. Sometimes, if where I am has a better, appropriate meal, I eat it and save mine for another time. It will always stay fresh and cold in my cooler. I am coming up on 10 months of this and I am down 120 pounds!

> "I wore a size 24 at our first meeting. I wore a size 10 to our most recent meeting and am still losing. I am much more active now and it goes without saying how truly wonderful I feel.
>
> "I owe it all to being prepared!"

Anywhere Visualizations

Whenever you have a rough day or moment—one of those times when you're feeling stressed or depressed or particularly vulnerable—turn to these visualizations for help. They will give you the internal drive you need to remain steadfast in your goals.

I've always believed in the power of visualization. The saying "what you see is what you get" applies. When you create a positive mental picture in your mind, you set off a series of events that help to create that picture in reality. So cultivate the image of a healthier, happier, trimmer you and you'll be well on your way to 3-Hour Diet™ success!

Visualization 1

Today you are going to take a journey one year into the future. Close your eyes and take a few deep, relaxing breaths.

You are getting ready to attend a wedding for your best friend, and you are the maid or matron of honor or best man! See yourself pull the long, slinky dress out of your closet or admire your tuxedo. Drape your clothes over a chair and take a good look. How do you think you will look all dressed up for the special event? How do you think it will feel on your now-slimmer body?

Pull on your clothes and feel the fabric fall around your body. Notice how your dress or tuxedo feels, how no part of it bunches or grabs. It fits perfectly. Notice your slender arms and how shapely your shoulders are. Turn around and take in your rear view. How do you look? How do you feel?

Now, see yourself a few hours later, dancing at the wedding reception. Notice how all eyes are on you, admiring how you look. See a smile creep across your face. You've reached your goal and you look fantastic.

Visualization 2

Today you are going to see yourself at your goal weight, a few years in the future. Today is the day of your high school class reunion. You haven't seen most of your classmates in many, many years. You are excited to show off what has become of you—how slim, healthy, and happy you are! It's time to get dressed. Imagine what you are wearing. What shoes do you slip on your feet? What jewelry do you put on? How do you style your hair? What makeup do you apply? How do you feel when you look in the mirror? You look great and feel fabulous!

As you approach the entrance of the reunion, take a deep breath and then confidently glide into the room. Whom do you see from high school and what do they say to you? Hear the compliments and "oohs" and "ahs." Tell your classmates how terrific you feel. Later in the evening, a class picture is taken. See yourself, standing tall, lean, and confident among your high school classmates.

Visualization 3

It's time to get dressed up in your finest attire because tonight you are going to shine at a very elegant, formal affair! You are going to wear that little black dress, the one you've kept in the back of your closet for when you had a body to show off. So, close your eyes and take a few relaxing breaths, in through your nose and out through your mouth.

See yourself getting ready for your special occasion. See the black dress hanging in your closet. Walk over to it. Take it out of the closet and drape it over the front of your body. Feel yourself growing excited at the prospect of finally wearing the dress. Lay the dress on your bed and notice every detail about it. Think back to the last time you wore it. How long ago was that? Then pick it up and slip it on. Feel the silky material fall evenly over your body. Put on your shoes and take a look at yourself in the mirror.

See your belly, how nothing bulges. See your slender, toned arms. Then, fast-forward to your big event. See yourself in the ballroom. Sense all of the eyes on you. You are confident and stunning. Dance the night away and enjoy it!

Visualization 4

Today is a glorious summer day filled with sunshine and warm breezes. It's the perfect day to hit the beach. Close your eyes and take a few relaxing breaths, in through your nose and out through your mouth.

You've just gotten off the phone with your friend and you've decided to go spend the day at the beach. You haven't been to the beach in many years, ever since you became too embarrassed to wear a swimsuit in public. But now you've got a beautiful body. So slip on your swimsuit, flip-flops, and wide-brimmed straw hat. You and your friend sing along to oldies music on the way to the beach. Once there, you sink your toes into the hot sand and let out a deep sigh of delight. Doesn't it feel great? As you spread out on your towel, you feel confident and beautiful. Feel the warm rays on your back and give your friend a wink. She comments on how great you look and you reply with a heartfelt "thank you" and tell her just how great you feel. The two of you spend the afternoon gossiping, frolicking in the waves, and strolling the length of the water's edge.

Visualization 5

Close your eyes and take a few relaxing breaths—in through your nose and out through your mouth. Smile and jump into the future with me.

I want you to visualize yourself after you've reached your goal. Notice your entire body. See how fit and firm your arms have become. Notice your vibrant skin. Visualize how your clothes will fall on your body and how your shoes will fit. Imagine the colors, the textures, and the patterns of a favorite outfit that you will be wearing. What does the new you look like? Will you have a new haircut, new look, or new accessories? See your body doing different movements. See yourself walking, sitting at work, or driving in your car. Try to visualize every detail. You've got to smell, hear, touch, and taste your vision to make it a reality.

Visualization 6

Close your eyes and take a few relaxing breaths—in through your nose and out through your mouth. Smile and jump into the future with me. Visualize the day that you reach your goal.

See yourself jump out of bed. As you get dressed, notice how you look. See your new sexy arms, legs, and torso. Go ahead and get dressed, making sure to pick that outfit you've always wanted to wear, but couldn't because of your weight. Notice how your clothes drape loosely over your body. Feel how none of the fabric hugs you or feels tight. Touch your body with your hands. How does it feel? Walk around. Notice that your thighs no longer rub together.

Look in the mirror and see how extraordinary

you look and feel. What quality about your new self are you most proud of?

Smile. You've reached your goal!

How to Drink Alcohol

Many clients ask me how to incorporate drinking into their 3-Hour Diet™ lifestyle. Although we recommend that you limit your alcohol intake while on the 3-Hour-Diet™, we have created options for you if, on occasion, you have more than one glass. Choose either option A or B below. Option A allows you to replace your evening treat with one drink and option B allows more than one drink if you follow the "drink reserve" guidelines one page 150.

Option A:

If you feel like having a drink with your dinner in the evening, make it your treat, but be sure it fits the program. Some ideas:

1. Make a 3-Hour Diet™–approved Wine Spritzer. Check the chart on page 144 for tips on how to mix it.

2. Make a 3-Hour Diet™–approved cocktail such as a Seven

and Seven with diet soda or Rum and Diet Coke in place of your evening treat. These two are slightly more than 50 calories, but close enough for a thumbs-up. Check the chart on page 144 for tips on how to mix them.

Option B:

If you want to drink more than offered in Option A, use these 3 steps:

- STEP 1: Set your drink count before you go out.

- STEP 2: Burn the calories before you head out. You've gotta burn extra calories in anticipation of consuming extra calories. That's the secret. See the chart How to Create a Drink Reserve on page 150 to decide how much exercise you need.

- STEP 3: Enjoy yourself!

Note: *Watch out for some popular favorites! A 5-ounce Margarita packs a walloping 340 calories! A very cool 4-ounce Cosmopolitan will add 250 calories to your day. You can have them, but you'll need to do more exercise to burn those extra calories.*

50—Calorie Treat Drinks

Wine Spritzer	2½ ounces wine (50 calories)
	6 ounces seltzer or Diet 7 UP® (0 calories)
Rum and Diet Coke	1 ounce spiced rum (60 calories)
	4 ounces Diet Coke® (0 calories)
	Twist of lime (freebie)
Seven and Diet Seven	1 ounce whiskey (60 calories)
	8 ounces diet lemon-lime soda (0 calories)
	Twist of lime (freebie)
Cherry Bomb Vodka	1 ounce UV Cherry Vodka (60 calories)

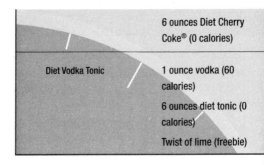

6 ounces Diet Cherry Coke® (0 calories)

Diet Vodka Tonic

1 ounce vodka (60 calories)

6 ounces diet tonic (0 calories)

Twist of lime (freebie)

Mixing the perfect 3-Hour Diet ™–Approved Cocktail

The previous chart contains some favorite cocktails with recipes to help you stay on the program while enjoying yourself. There are a few that stay in the 50-calorie range; you can have one of these in place of a treat in the evening. All of the others are approximately 100 calories, which is the amount burned with each of the *Burners* I've listed on page 150. Remember, a standard shot glass measures 1½ ounces.

100-Calorie Cocktails

Light Beer— they vary, so make sure to check the label.	12 ounces (one regular size can or bottle)
Miller Lite	
Amstel® Light	
Aspen Edge ™	
Natural Light	
Michelob® ULTRA (95 cal)	
Coors Light (102 cal)	
Bud Light	
Bud Ice Light®	
Busch Light® (110 cal)	
Red or white wine (no port/dessert wine)	5 ounces (100 calories)
Vodka Tonic	1 ounce vodka (60 calories)
	4 ounces tonic (40 calories)
	Twist of lime (freebie)

Bloody Mary	1½ ounces vodka (90 calories)
	4 ounces/½ cup tomato juice (20 calories)
	Lime twist
	dash Tabasco®
	dash pepper
	dash Worcestershire (freebies)
	1 celery stick (freebie)
Gin and Tonic	1 ounce gin (60 calories)
	4 ounces tonic (40 calories)
	Twist of lime (freebie)
Gimlet	1½ ounces gin or vodka (90 calories)
	½ ounce sweetened lime juice (4 calories)
	Twist of lime (freebie)

Bloody Maria	1½ ounces tequila (90 calories)
	4 ounces/½ cup tomato juice (20 calories)
	Lemon twist
	dash Tabasco®
	dash salt (freebies)
Rum and Coke®	1 ounce spiced rum (60 calories)
	4 ounces Coca-Cola® (48 calories)
	Twist of lime (freebie)
Seven and Seven	1 ounce whiskey (60 calories)
	2 ounces regular lemon-lime soda (28 calories)
	6 ounces diet lemon-lime soda (0 calories)
	Twist of lime (freebie)

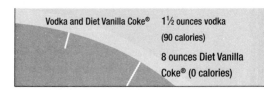

Vodka and Diet Vanilla Coke®   1½ ounces vodka
                                (90 calories)

                                8 ounces Diet Vanilla
                                Coke® (0 calories)

More tips for drinking alcohol on the 3-Hour Diet™

- Remember that serving size is key. If you're not making the drink, be specific with the bartender.

- The proof makes a difference with hard alcohol, so check the bottle. The calorie counts provided in my charts are based on 80-proof; the higher the proof, the higher the calorie count.

- Use the calorie amounts of the different alcoholic drinks on the previous pages to create other suitable 50- and 100-calorie drinks you might like. If you like having a shot, that's fine, just remember the calories still count, and keep track!

How to Create a Drink Reserve

Below you'll find some activities to help you burn off those 100-calorie cocktails. Remember, I don't recommend drinking too much while trying to lose weight, but if you are going to have more than one drink, complete one of the activities below to create the "drink reserve." You have to multiply how long you do the activity by how many drinks you plan to have. If you decide to splurge on a higher-calorie drink, you'll have to exercise more to balance it out.

Burners (each one creates a 100-calorie reserve)	How Long
Walking 3 mph	19 Minutes
Jogging 5 mph	11 Minutes
Energetic dancing	14 Minutes
Active aerobics	12 Minutes
Biking	12 Minutes
Steady swimming	11 Minutes

Vigorous housecleaning (floor scrubbing, vacuuming, sweeping)	20 Minutes
Gardening (raking, mowing, squatting to pull weeds)	15 Minutes
Washing car	20 Minutes

No-Calorie and Low-Calorie Drink Options

No-Calorie Options

All these drinks have no calories. They are a perfect combination with any one of your lunch or dinner choices.

Penta®

Penta® Water 16.9 ounces

Penta® Water 1 liter

Note: Jorge recommends this water to all his clients due to its extremely high purity. Your goal is to have 8 glasses of water each day.

Coca-Cola® Products

Coca-Cola® zero™

Diet Coke®

Caffeine-free Diet Coke®

Diet Coke® Sweetened with Splenda®

Diet Coke® with Lime

Diet Coke® with Lemon

Diet Cherry Coke®

Fresca®

Diet INCA KOLA®

Diet Sprite Zero®

TaB®

Diet Vanilla Coke®

Diet Barq's® Root Beer

Diet Barq's® Vanilla Cream

Diet Mello Yello®

Diet Northern Neck® Ginger Ale

Nestea® Diet Lemon

Nestea® Unsweetened

Diet Nestea® COOL

Seagram's® Diet Ginger Ale

Seagram's® Diet Raspberry Ginger Ale

Seagram's® Club Soda

Seagram's® Diet Tonic Water

Seagram's® Lemon Lime Seltzer Naturals

Seagram's® Orange Seltzer Naturals

Seagram's® Black Cherry Seltzer Naturals

Seagram's® Raspberry Seltzer Naturals

Seagram's® Original Seltzer

Seagram's® Sparkling Water

Pepsi-Cola® Products

Diet Pepsi®

Diet Caffeine Free Pepsi®

Diet Pepsi® Twist

Diet Pepsi® Vanilla

Diet Wild Cherry Pepsi®

Pepsi® ONE

Diet Lipton® Brisk Lemon Flavored

Diet Mountain Dew® Code Red®

Diet Mountain Dew®

Diet Caffeine-Free Mountain Dew®

Diet Mug® Root Beer

Diet Mug® Cream Soda

Sierra Mist® Free

Diet Orange Slice

Tropicana® Sugar Free Lemonade

Tropicana® Sugar Free Fruit Punch

Tropicana® Sugar Free Orangeade

SoBe® Lean® Diet Cranberry Grapefruit

SoBe® Lean® Energy Diet Citrus

SoBe® Lean® Diet Green Tea

SoBe® Lean® Diet Mango Melon

SoBe® Lean® Diet Peach Tea

Hansen's®

Hansen's® Diet Soda Tangerine Lime

Hansen's® Diet Soda Peach

Hansen's® Diet Soda Kiwi Strawberry

Hansen's® Diet Soda Ginger Ale

Hansen's® Diet Soda Creamy Root Beer

Hansen's® Diet Soda Black Cherry

RC® COLA

Diet Rite® Red Raspberry

Diet Rite® Tangerine

Diet Rite® White Grape

Diet Rite® Cola

Diet Rite® Kiwi Strawberry

Diet Rite® Black Cherry

Diet Royal Crown RC® Cola

Diet Vernors® Ginger Soda

Polar® Beverages

Polar® Diet Birch Beer

Polar® Diet Black Cherry

Polar® Diet Cola

Polar® Diet Cream Soda

Polar® Diet Double Fudge

Polar® Diet Grape

Polar® Diet Lemon Lime

Polar® Diet Orange Dry

Polar® Diet Raspberry Ginger Ale

Polar® Diet Raspberry Lime

Polar® Diet Root Beer

Polar® Diet Strawberry

Arizona®

Arizona® Black Tea, Diet Lemon Tea
Arizona® Black Tea, Diet Peach Tea
Arizona® Black Tea, Diet Raspberry Tea
Arizona® Green Tea, Diet Green Tea

Dr Pepper/7 UP® Products

Diet Sunkist®
Diet 7 UP®
Diet A&W® Root Beer

Low-Calorie Options

The following drinks are low in calories; 5–10 calories per serving. They are not unlimited like the no-calorie drinks above, but can be consumed in moderation.

Crystal Light®

Crystal Light® Raspberry Ice
Crystal Light® Pink Lemonade
Crystal Light® Lemonade
Crystal Light® Lemon Tea
Crystal Light® Strawberry Kiwi

FUZE®

FUZE® slenderize, Cranberry Raspberry
FUZE® slenderize, Cranberry Apple
FUZE® slenderize, Tropical Punch

Hansen's®

Hansen's® Energy Water E_2O™, Tangerine
Hansen's® Energy Water E_2O™, Lemon
Hansen's® Energy Water E_2O™, Apple
Hansen's® Energy Water E_2O™, Berry
Hansen's® Diet Red Energy®

Minute Maid® Light™ Guava Citrus
Minute Maid® Light™ Mango Tropical

Eating at Events

Living a healthy lifestyle shouldn't mean skipping out on the fun! You can still attend those events you've always enjoyed; you just need to have a plan in place to be sure you don't overindulge on food when you're indulging your active side. Try these tips:

BBQ or Ball Game

Some favorites that won't leave you striking out:

- 1 hamburger with half the bun and ½ cup of pasta salad.

- 3 ribs, corn, and green salad with low-fat dressing.

- Grilled chicken without skin, rice or mashed potatoes, and grilled veggies or fruit salad.

- Reduced-fat hot dog, green salad with a squeeze of lemon, and a small roll or half the bun.

- Turkey burger (patty only), french fries, and a Caesar salad with lemon for dressing.

If you're heading to a BBQ with friends, don't be afraid to bring your own grilling selection. Friends will understand that you're making a concerted effort to be healthy and will support your efforts. You can always sample their green or fruit salad sides or have half of one of their homemade cookies as your treat.

Wedding Event

The happy couple will say "I do," but a few "no, thanks" on your part can keep you on track. Make the following smart choices in order to keep your own vow:

- Grilled fish, rice, and vegetables. Skip any heavy sauces and season the fish with fresh lemon.

- Chicken, pasta, and salad. Chicken is pretty standard wedding fare. Keep the pasta to a ½-cup serving and watch the salad dressing. Get it on the side and ask for a light option.

- Scallops with broccoli, salad, and a wheat roll. Any salad will do, but skip the butter on your roll if you're having dressing.

- Omelet with spinach, tomatoes, and potatoes. Ask for egg whites if possible, and keep it to a two-egg omelet if it's whole eggs.

- Sliced roast beef, potato, and green salad. Be careful with creamy sauces and toppings on the potato—you want to have a few calories left for some cake.

- When the cake is served, try two bites and then hit the dance floor!

Parties of All Occasions

Fend off the fried stuff, banish the brie, and picture how great you'll look in your outfit by trying these suggestions at the next cocktail soiree:

- Bruschetta. Small pieces of bread and lots of fresh tomatoes are a tasty treat!

- Fresh veggies and low-cal dip. Focus on the veggies; you can't overdo those.

- Grilled chicken skewers.

- Sushi.

- Turkey wrap rolls. Watch out for heavy spreads: keep them to a minimum if they're covered in mayo.

- Shrimp with cocktail sauce.

- Cheese and crackers. These can add up quickly. Remember to keep your cheese consumption to about the size of two dice.

- Mini quiche. Hold yourself to just a couple of bite-size pieces!

Remember, if the appetizers are your main meal, you can have a bite-size sample of each thing and feel good about your 3-Hour Plate.™ Look for grilled chicken skewers, shrimp or turkey wraps to get enough protein, and go heavy on the veggies. If dinner is to follow, stick to the veggies and save up for the main attraction!

Don't forget to drink lots of water so you stay hydrated and filled up!

THE 3-HOUR DIET™ ADDITIONAL TOOLS

Want to get the most out of the 3-Hour Diet™? Check out these ways to take your plan to the next level.

3-HOUR DIET™ ONLINE

Join the **3HourDiet.net** online center and keep your taste buds excited with even more delicious ideas for on-the-go eating and easy home cooking!

Join our club and you'll get:

1. A personalized, printable weekly 3-hour meal planner
2. Delicious recipes you can make in minutes
3. Frozen-food options from brand names like Lean Cuisine®, Healthy Choice®, Amy's®
4. Fast-food options from: McDonald's®, KFC®, Arby's®, Subway®, In 'N' Out®, Taco Bell®, Burger King®, Jack in the Box®, and many more

Plus you get access to our Jorge support boards, online meetings, and a buddy system.

For a free tour of the 3-Hour Diet™ Online, go to 3HourDiet.net today.

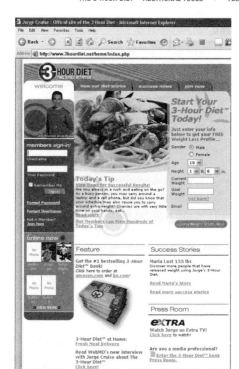

MORE SUPPORT TOOLS

The 3-Hour Diet™ At Home Fresh Delivery

Take all the thinking out of following the 3-Hour Diet™ eating plan. Imagine receiving three delicious chef-prepared meals, two snacks, and one delicious treat delivered fresh to your door. Visit *3HourDietAtHome.com* to live like a star today.

The 3-Hour Diet™ Original Book

This is the book that started the revolution. A must for anyone who wants all the secrets to the 3-Hour Diet™. Includes more than 50 easy recipes, in-depth success stories, and an insider's look at fad diets, including how low-carb diets make you fat. Available everywhere books are sold.

The 3-Hour Diet™ Audio Book

Experience the 3-Hour Diet™ revolution direct from Jorge Cruise. On his exclusive audio program he will walk you through all the secrets of how to lose 2 pounds a week without any deprivation or fad dieting. As an added bonus you will also hear actual success interviews with 3-Hour Diet™ clients. Get ready to boost your motivation and success to the highest levels! Available everywhere books are sold.

The 3-Hour Diet™ Book in Spanish

Jorge's edition in Spanish has an inspirational foreword written by TV talks-how host Cristina from *El Show de Cristina*. This version is perfect for the Spanish-speaking loved one in your life. Available everywhere books are sold.

8 Minutes in the Morning® Book Series

Want to accelerate your results? Then make sure to get Jorge's exercise book series. These toning and firming exercises are used at home to restore lost muscle, thus revving your metabolism even higher. And they only take 8 minutes a day! Available everywhere books are sold.

AOL Diet Coach

Jorge Cruise is AOL's exclusive Diet Coach. Visit AOL.com for exclusive interactive material from Jorge to keep you looking and feeling your best.

USA WEEKEND

Visit usaweekend.com for each new "Fit-smart" article Jorge writes as a contributing columnist for *USA WEEKEND* magazine. Also get access to his past archives.

First for Women Magazine

Every issue Jorge answers your questions in his advice column. Available in your supermarket checkout lines everywhere.

Extra TV

Every month Jorge interviews America's top Hollywood TV and movie stars to find out what they are eating to look camera-ready. Visit ExtraTV.com for more details and air times.

JORGE CRUISE'S BIOGRAPHY

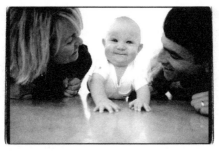

The Cruise family: Heather, Parker, and Jorge

Jorge Cruise personally struggled with weight as a child and young man. Today he is recognized as America's leading weight-loss expert for busy people. He is the *New York Times* best-selling author of *8 Minutes in the Morning*® (published in 14 languages) and the author of the new best seller *The 3-Hour Diet™*. Jorge has also coached more than 3 million online clients at 3hourdiet.net and is the exclusive "Diet Coach" for AOL's 23 million subscribers. Jorge is seen nationwide as the regular "Diet & Fitness Correspondent" for *Extra* and serves as the "Slimming Coach" for *First for Women* magazine. More than 50 million *USA WEEKEND* readers enjoy timely advice from Jorge as their regular "FitSmart Columnist," and in addition, Jorge appears regularly on television shows that include *Oprah, Good Morning America, The Today Show, Dateline* NBC, CNN and *The View*. He can be contacted at JorgeCruise.com.

> "Jorge Cruise has answers that really work and take almost no time.
> I recommend them highly."
>
> **—ANDREW WEIL, MD,**
> Director of the Program
> in Integrative Medicine,
> University of Arizona

Visit 3HourDiet.net for your FREE personalized weight-loss profile.

INDEX